WHAT YOU NEED TO KNOW ABOUT PROZAC AND THE NEW ANTIDEPRESSANTS

More than 11 million people worldwide are currently taking Prozac, but what do most of these people really know about this so-called miracle drug and the other new antidepressants being prescribed? This comprehensive look at each of these drugs and their pros and cons answers such questions as:

- Will Prozac make me lose the essence of my personality or make me out of control?
- Can I take other drugs along with Prozac?
- Are these drugs addictive?
- What are the side effects, and how can I manage them?
- And much more

WILLIAM S. APPLETON, M.D., is a psychiatrist with his own private practice and is on the faculty at Harvard Medical School. The author of several books, he has appeared on more than 120 television and radio shows. He lives in Cambridge, Massachusetts.

Other Books by William Appleton, M.D.

Practical Clinical Psychopharmacology, 3rd Edition
The Fifth Psychoactive Drug Usage Guide

PROZAC

AND THE

NEW ANTIDEPRESSANTS

WHAT YOU NEED TO KNOW ABOUT PROZAC, ZOLOFT, PAXIL, LUVOX, WELLBUTRIN, EFFEXOR, SERZONE, AND MORE

William S. Appleton, M.D.

A PLUME BOOK

PUBLISHER'S NOTE
The ideas, procedures, and suggestions contained in this book are not intended as a
substitute for consulting with your physician. All matters regarding your health require
medical supervision.

PLUME
Published by the Penguin Group
Penguin Books USA Inc., 375 Hudson Street, New York, New York 10014, U.S.A.
Penguin Books Ltd, 27 Wrights Lane, London W8 5TZ, England
Penguin Books Australia Ltd, Ringwood, Victoria, Australia
Penguin Books Canada Ltd, 10 Alcorn Avenue, Toronto, Ontario, Canada M4V 3B2
Penguin Books (N.Z.) Ltd, 182-190 Wairau Road, Auckland 10, New Zealand

Penguin Books Ltd, Registered Offices:
Harmondsworth, Middlesex, England

First published by Plume, an imprint of Dutton Signet,
a division of Penguin Books USA Inc.

First Printing, January, 1997
10 9 8 7 6 5 4 3

LIBRARY OF CONGRESS CATALOGING-IN-PUBLICATION DATA:

Appleton, William S.
    Prozac and the new antidepressants : what you need to know about prozac, zoloft,
paxil, wellbutrin, effexor, serzone, luvox, and more / William S. Appleton.
        p.   cm.
    Includes bibliographical references and index.
    ISBN 0-452-27443-5
    1. Serotonin uptake inhibitors—Popular works. 2. Antidepressants—Popular works.
I. Title.
    RM332.A67   1997
    616.85'2706—dc20   96–27541
                                                            CIP

Printed in the United States of America
Set in New Baskerville
Designed by Leonard Telesca

To the memory of
Gerald L. Klerman, M.D.

Contents

Acknowledgments

I wish to thank my editor, Deborah Brody, whose idea inspired this book and whose kind, firm hand guided me. Thanks also to Lindy Hess, my wife, who edits me on a daily basis. I am especially grateful to my colleagues at the Massachusetts Mental Health Center, who have taught me most of what I know about psychiatric drugs, psychotherapy, and taking care of patients. Thanks to Karen Wood for deciphering my handwriting and entering it into the computer, and to Beth Banov, librarian, and Anne Dantzler, M.D.

Author's Note

The dosages and indications of the drugs in this book conform to the standards of the U.S. Food and Drug Administration and the practices of the general medical community. However, the usage of some of the medications in certain conditions may not have specific FDA approval. Because therapeutic standards continually change, especially with drugs as new as those described here, it is necessary for readers to have their treatment supervised by a physician directly involved in their care.

Prozac + new anti depressants

RW 332.A67

Before Prozac

RC 534.552

INTRODUCTION

If you've picked up this book, chances are that you (or someone you care about) suffer from depression and are considering taking an antidepressant. You've probably heard about Prozac and the other new antidepressants—the so-called wonder drugs used to treat depression—and you're trying to figure out if you are a good candidate for taking one. This book will help you make that decision. It describes in detail how these drugs work, tells you the advantages and disadvantages of each, explains each drug's side effects, and compares the various drugs to each other.

Why Are Most Depressed People Not Treated With an Antidepressant?

A 1992 study found that only 11 percent of those needing an antidepressant drug get it. While the headlines have it that we live in a "Prozac Nation," the fact is, for a variety of reasons, most depressed people are *not* treated. One reason is the belief that psychiatric illness is due to lack of moral strength and that whatever the problem, one needs to go it alone. Except for the severely depressed (and even their plight is often overlooked), most people who suffer from a more mild depression drag themselves through work and collapse at home without realizing that something is wrong. More often than not, their doctors treat them for fatigue, insomnia, indigestion, and/or backache—or not at all—rather than for the underlying depression. With both the patient and the doctor unwilling to admit or simply unaware of the true nature of the illness, it is little wonder that depression goes untreated. But even when the patient and/or doctor is aware of the illness, there are other factors conspiring against adequate help. In the minds of many people who suffer from depression, taking medication means admitting one is sick, and furthermore, that it is serious. Some are more willing to accept "talk therapy" because it implies a milder condition. In addition, the depression itself blocks the expectation of treatment. The illness, which is accompanied by diminished energy, indecisiveness, guilt, feelings of worthlessness, and loss of hope, destroys the notion of relief. It makes the sufferer unable to mobilize and take action to seek help. It is my hope that this book will make you aware that being depressed is not the way life is or need be, and that you may have an illness for which there is safe, effective, and rapid treatment.

Getting Help

Once you have decided that you have a clinical depression in need of treatment, the first thing you need to do is get professional help. Since this is a book on the new antidepressants available, I will concentrate on them, but for most depressed patients, psychotherapy is equally important. While my discussion of psychotherapy will be necessarily brief, it is important that anyone seeking treatment for depression have a good idea of what help to expect from drugs and what issues require talk therapy, for it is in the combination of the two that the best hope lies.

The first step in getting help is to find a good therapist. Physicians, clergy, friends, and relatives can be excellent sources for a recommendation. If none of these are available, try the local medical or psychiatric society or a nearby medical school. Consider your first visit a trial in which you evaluate what is said to you and whether you feel comfortable with the person you see. It is essential not only that you like the therapist, but that they impress you with their capacity to understand your situation and have something helpful to tell you. If the therapist is not a physician and you require an antidepressant, then either your own doctor or a psychiatrist will have to prescribe it. Once this is done, it is essential that the therapist and the doctor who prescribed the medication confer regularly about your progress. If you are already in psychotherapy with a nonphysician and also wish to try an antidepressant, discuss it with your therapist. Most will welcome the possibility of adding medication to ease your pain, but a minority may accuse you of dodging responsibility and seeking an easy way out. This minority does not understand that psychotherapy and antidepressants work better together for depressed people than either does alone.

The chapters that follow discuss what depression is, how it is treated, and describe the groups of drugs that are being widely used to treat it. It is my hope that this book will help you find the answers you are looking for and start you on the road to a happier, healthier life.

CHAPTER 1

Understanding Major Depression

Before discussing the new antidepressants in detail, it is important to understand exactly what depression is and how it is diagnosed. This chapter takes you step-by-step through the symptoms and diagnosis of major depression.

The Symptoms of a Major Depressive Episode

Although the term *clinical depression* is commonly used, the precise term is *major depression*, which is what I will use throughout this book. The symptoms of major depression are the following:

Depressed Mood

A depressed mood is a constant sad, dejected feeling lasting at least two weeks, which must be differentiated from normal blues or discouragement. Although the difference between feeling sad and depression can be hard to distinguish in words, those who have experienced both have little difficulty in telling them apart.

Hopelessness is central to this mood, a feeling that there is nothing to look forward to and that the pain will never cease. This desperate, miserable feeling can be accompanied by excessive worry about anything or everything, including money, health, family, work, and friendships.

A depressed mood can be the most painful affliction a human can suffer. Depressed patients who break a leg or get pneumonia welcome the physical pain as a distraction from their extreme psychological discomfort. Their gloomy pessimism allows them no hope of escape from their agony. They do not expect to get well.

Depressed people may find themselves bursting into tears without warning. They may run from the sight of others, embarrassed by their loss of control.

Being in a depressed mood can make one excessively sensitive and "thin-skinned," quick to take offense, easily hurt and discouraged. The depressed person can overreact to his own errors and therefore be unwilling to take chances and try new or difficult tasks. At work, depressives are timid, afraid to be inventive, and most comfortable with routine assignments.

Depressives can be irritable, and some are subject to sudden rages. They are often short on patience and bristle for little or no reason.

The mood of the depressive may or may not be influenced by actual events. Some are highly reactive, instantly lifted by praise or thrown to the depths by criticism. Such individuals are viewed by friends and colleagues as requiring very careful handling. People walk on eggshells around them. The insensitive spouse has no recognition of how much he influences his depressive partner's mood. One thoughtless boss's praise and criticism caused his depressed assistant to go from joy to gloom because of her exquisite sensitivity. Other depressives show little reaction to the good things that happen to them. In fact, they seem only to register the bad, particularly the slights and criticisms they encounter. Some experts have judged the unreactive depressives to be more severe, but it may be that they are just different. If a patient were to commit suicide in reaction to rejection, to call such a depression less severe makes no sense.

The pain of the depressed mood makes the sufferer seek relief in a large variety of actions, ranging from harmless to life-threatening. The unhappy go shopping, take a vacation, change jobs, careers, even spouses, while the acutely tormented drink too much, take drugs, or induce pain by relentlessly picking at their fingers or cutting themselves in an attempt to relieve the pain in their head.

A depressed mood often influences the way a depressive relates to others. Some seek out friends and loved ones in an effort to feel better by interacting with others. The pain of their illness makes them more dependent on others. They call their friends and relatives incessantly on the phone, require their spouse to listen to them endlessly, and wear everyone out with inordinate demands on their time. Often their complaints and concerns are dull and repetitious. Some seem to ask for advice, which they then ignore, frustrating those giving it. Such people feel much worse when alone. Others seek solitude and find being with people a strain— false and meaningless. They hide when depressed, call no one, do not answer their phone, and, when forced to communicate with others, do so monosyllabically.

Loss of Interest or Pleasure in Activities

When loss of interest or pleasure in activities is sudden and all-inclusive, it is easy for the patient, the family, and the doctor to recognize. For example, a previously lively and involved working mother stops caring about her job or children, and only wants to stay in bed and do nothing. She is clearly experiencing a decline of interest and pleasure in her usual activities. When the change is more gradual and selective in its targets, it can be more difficult to evaluate. For example, the loss of satisfaction may initially be limited to responsibilities and obligations, while the desire for recreational activities and vacations increases. A woman may say she hates her job or even her husband, but will continue to enjoy long lunches or trips to Europe. A student may stop studying or going to class, but will spend time skiing and partying. The person who says that being a lawyer or shopkeeper is no longer interesting is often depressed rather than merely ready for a career change. When a man says he no longer loves his wife of seventeen years, he may hide the underlying depressive cause of his loss of pleasure in her company in seemingly normal-sounding phrases, such as "we have grown apart," "she is immature," "she only cares about clothes and appearances." Many depressions are missed by the patient, the family, and even the doctor because they are described in terms that seem understandable and not pathological. Before you change your job or spouse, find out whether your misery is due to a major depression rather than circumstances outside you. The distinction between internally and externally caused depression can be difficult and may require the help of a psychiatrist.

The loss of interest and pleasure affects one's ability to plan for the future, especially long-term. This absence of spontaneous motivation means the sufferer will do only that which he or she is forced to do, either by necessity or by an employer. This condition has been described as a paralysis of will, in which the point of doing anything at all seems lost. Goals that once attracted—the desire for money, fame, prestige, success—no longer seem worthwhile. The notion that "there is no point" and that "life is futile" takes over in the absence of pleasure.

In the deepest depressions, when all interest and pleasure is gone, the sufferer has no desire to do anything. There is no gratification from food or sex. Psychiatrists take the inability to work and the cessation of all sexual desire as signs of the deepest depression, requiring prompt and rigorous treatment.

Can You Be Depressed Without a Depressed Mood?

To be diagnosed as having a depression you must be suffering from *either* a depressed mood *or* a loss of interest and pleasure in usual activities, but not necessarily both. How can someone be depressed without a depressed mood? Sometimes it is because the person does not recognize the mood or will not admit to it. Those who consider depression to have the stigma of mental illness fight the recognition. Others consider long periods of low mood to be a normal part of life for which there is no diagnosis or treatment. Some patients do not complain of sadness but appear depressed, and occasionally will admit it when others point it out. Major depressives may suffer severe aches and pains in the stomach, back, or head, but do not say they feel unhappy. These bodily equivalents of the mental pain associated with a depressed mood often respond to antidepressant drug therapies. Patients with major depressive disorder can suffer from other aspects of the illness but not from a depressed mood. They may tell their friends, family, even their doctors that they cannot sleep, have severe headaches or stomachaches, that they are exhausted, but not that they have a depressed mood. It is up to the doctor to recognize and treat such people for depression. Unfortunately, the diagnosis is often missed. One study found that over 70 percent of such patients were not diagnosed by their medical doctors as depressed when they should have been, and thus they underwent many unnecessary tests for physical illness and failed to be relieved of their depression.

Bodily Changes

Changes in weight, sleep patterns, activity, and energy levels are characteristic of major depression.

Weight

Although weight and appetite may be significantly increased

or decreased, the most typical pattern is that of weight loss accompanied by little desire for food. The depressed patient may lose 5 percent of his or her body weight within a month without dieting. This can be alarming and may trigger a medical workup to make sure an organic illness is not the cause. Less severely depressed patients may eat too much. Some say food is comforting and makes them feel better, while others have cravings for sweets and other high-caloric foods. One such woman gained fifty pounds in one year.

Sleep

The most typical major depressive sleep disturbance involves awakening in the middle of the night and finding it very difficult or impossible to go back to sleep. The patient's day may begin at three or four in the morning, making him or her appear and feel exhausted. In addition, the depressive may also have trouble falling asleep. A minority of depressives sleep too much, finding their only pleasure in escaping from the world. One woman would do only what she had to do for the care of her family and otherwise spent most of her life in bed. She could think of nothing more enjoyable to do with her time. But most depressives complain constantly of their inability to sleep. They dread getting into bed and facing another long sleepless night. They beg for sleeping pills to help them rest.

Activity

There are two types of activity changes occurring in major depressives: agitation and retardation. Agitation is a state of constant restless motion which in major depressives can take the form of pacing aimlessly, hand-wringing, and being unable to sit still. For purposes of formal diagnosis, the condition must be severe enough so that the agitation is noticeable to others. Retardation, also objectively observable, is evident in movement and in speech. There is a slowing of thought and verbal response. The patient has almost nothing to say spontaneously and answers questions monosyllabically or not at all. Such a person is boring to be with and hard to talk to.

Energy

A depressed person with low energy may awaken tired or become easily wearied by normal physical or mental effort. Even previously simple tasks seem a burden. Letters remain unanswered, even unopened, while routine tasks take longer. Anything new or out of the ordinary is avoided. This loss of energy may be wrongly attributed to physical illness, and a series of expensive medical tests may be ordered. Or the patient may conclude that overwork is responsible and go on vacation, which provides temporary relief, but no permanent solution. Chronic fatigue syndrome can sometimes be due to unrecognized depression.

The seeming laziness of the depressed patient who appears unwilling to perform energetically either at work or at home can make employers and family extremely angry. If there were a physical cause, like pneumonia, others would be more forgiving. But depression is not a physical illness and the patient's loss of spontaneous motivation and movement can frustrate those around him because they do not understand the illness.

Thinking Changes

Thoughts of worthlessness or guilt, a diminished ability to think or concentrate, indecisiveness, and recurrent thoughts of death or suicide are also characteristics of major depression.

Sense of Worthlessness or Guilt

The overwhelming majority of depressed patients do not like themselves, denouncing themselves as inadequate in terms of all the qualities that they value: attractiveness, intelligence, and popularity. They feel ugly, stupid, unlovable, boring, and expect failure and rejection. They regard themselves as unequal to the tasks they attempt, and the more severely ill feel loathed by all who know them and deserving of severe punishment. No matter how successful they in fact are, they regard themselves as failures: millionaires feel poor, serious authors feel like hacks. But what of the average man and woman who say they have done nothing with their lives? Are they right? They fail to credit themselves with having taken care of their families, done careful, high-quality, and useful work, helped their communities and churches. Instead they see only what they have not done, castigating themselves as poor parents, bad citizens, and slipshod workers. They focus on failures, ignore successes, and are filled with self-reproaches and self-blame. Depending on the severity of the condition, the patient experiences anything from self-dislike to self-hatred. There is a great disparity between the person's self-image and objective fact.

Guilt overwhelms them: they believe they have done terrible things, caused others great harm, and should be punished. Excessively self-blaming, the depressed person feels responsible for anything that goes wrong. A mother whose son failed an exam in elementary school believed it was her fault for not making him study enough and in the right way. A man who could not earn enough money to indulge his family's most elaborate whim thought himself a failure rather than concluding that they spent too much. When committing a minor error, the depressed patient exaggerates both its magnitude and the terrible consequences it might produce. The depressed woman feels she deserves to suffer for her sins and is filled with self-reproaches and self-blame.

Diminished Ability to Think or Concentrate, or Indecisiveness

The depressed patient's capacity to think can be severely disturbed and seem like a demented person's inability to concentrate or remember. A student's grades may drop sharply and a worker's performance deteriorate completely. Indecisiveness can slow or totally disrupt a patient's ability to function. It is caused by an inability to concentrate and do the work of choosing among alternatives to pick a course of action, and by the expectation that things will not turn out well. In fact, indecisiveness is a by-product of several of the symptoms of depression: the inability to concentrate, the sense that one's efforts will never succeed, the tendency to become easily tired when attempting difficult tasks, the low self-esteem that makes the worker feel unequal to the task, and the slowing and poverty of thoughts and ideas. The depressed patient's IQ can test lower because of disturbance in concentration, failure in memory, fatigue, and loss of motivation. It is not just that the depressed patient feels unwell; it may indeed be that the brain works less well. But whether the ultimate cause is a disorder of mood or of thought or both, the damage to the person's performance is devastating.

Recurrent Thoughts of Death, Thoughts of or Attempts at Suicide

Severe depression can be a fatal disease in 5 to 15 percent of those who suffer from it. The pain of this illness makes thoughts of death or action to seek it seem a welcome relief. Many patients contemplating suicide keep their thoughts and plans to themselves. Those who speak of it openly should not be dismissed as mere attention-getters, but be taken seriously. Many suicide attempts fail not because the individual is merely seeking attention but because of poor planning at a time when the person is very upset. Friends and relatives must be aware of this danger and act to stop it. If you feel hopeless and are thinking of killing yourself to end your misery, you must understand that depression is a treatable disease and you can be helped.

Four Common Ways the Diagnosis of Major Depression Can Be Missed

The Pain Way

Donna is thirty-seven years old and living in a new city, having been transferred by her company. She works sixty hours a week and comes home to an empty apartment on a street of strangers. Her stomach has been bothering her for months now, and lately the pain keeps her up at night. She worries that she may have an ulcer or worse, and has made several appointments with her doctor, who, after prescribing antacids without success, has scheduled her for X rays to have a look at her stomach and intestines. The films have come back normal, and he recommends a psychiatric consultation. Donna agrees to go. Many people would not, offended that the doctor does not regard the pain as real. Donna worries that her medical doctor might think her crazy, but decides not to say anything about it. Her distress has made her willing to try anything.

Donna's psychiatric interview reveals a depressed mood, and feelings of sadness, loneliness, and boredom. These symptoms have occurred over the last several months as Donna was leaving her old job and starting her new one. She took little interest or pleasure in her daily life and forced herself through the workday, collapsing at home at the end. She has lost fifteen pounds in the last month and awakens in the middle of the night and finds herself unable to get back to sleep. Doing her job has become more and more of a chore. She finds it difficult to keep up with the mail or return phone calls and has little energy to go out on sales calls.

Donna, like many depressed people, experienced her main symptom in the form of pain. Some suffer headaches, others backaches, and many, like Donna, have abdominal disturbances. When busy medical doctors do not question these individuals for the other symptoms of depression, the diagnosis is often missed. Not all the fault of lack of proper treatment lies with hurried or careless doctors. Many patients are unwilling to go to a psychiatrist or to listen to their family physician's recommendations of treatment for depression. The stigma of mental illness prevents many sufferers from getting the help they need.

The Fatigue Way

Claire is fifty-two years old. Her children have left home and her job as a real estate agent has produced declining income for her. She wonders if it's the rising interest rates or increased competition, but she feels less inclined to work with the clients she has or to seek new ones. She finds her household chores more daunting and feels little inclination to cook for her husband when he comes home from work. She sits and watches television and lies around in bed. Her energy is so low that she has gone to several doctors to find out if her thyroid activity is low or if she is anemic. She even fears she may have some hidden cancer. But after numerous tests, nothing can be found. She becomes very angry when a psychiatric consultation is finally recommended. Her mother had been a serious depressive and Claire knows she is nothing like her. Perhaps she has chronic fatigue syndrome, but the possible viral cause cannot in her case be proved.

Unfortunately, Claire adamantly refuses psychiatric help. She is terrified she may have a version of her mother's depression. In fact, she does. She takes little interest or pleasure in her daily life, feels hopeless about her prospects for getting better, no longer enjoys sex with her husband, and feels anger toward him for requiring meals and her attention. She has difficulty falling asleep and awakens for long periods; sometimes she is unable to go back asleep at all. She looks tired and grim. Her thoughts have slowed and she makes little spontaneous conversation. It has been months since she could concentrate and read a book.

If you are fighting the recognition that you are depressed out of fear that you are crazy or morally defective, remember that depression is a painful illness for which there is effective treatment. You can be helped, but you must admit your need!

The Hate Way

John is a forty-one-year-old stockbroker who over the past year has come to hate his wife. He began to have affairs. Several times he thought he was in love with someone else, but each time would be drawn back home to try to make his marriage work, not only for the sake of the children but also because he believed in the preservation of the family. He did not like thinking of himself as just another midlife-crisis sufferer off chasing women. He would return and try, but he could not stand his wife. He thought her values superficial, that all she cared about was lunches with her friends and making social dates with other couples. He found her long rehashes of their socializing insufferable, and her desire to talk out their problems made him want to run away. He hated the way she made love to him, which he believed was motivated by her wish to hang on to him rather than by honest sexual desire. John pretended to participate in the couples therapies she would drag him to, but would find ways not to continue going.

The feeling "I no longer love my wife" is a common manifestation of major depression. John's depression makes him lose interest in, and derive no pleasure from, other people, including his wife, and the hatred caused by his mood disorder focuses on her. At the same time, his illness makes John very needy and he keeps returning to the wife he hates. The momentary antidepressant effect of his affairs cannot replace the comfort of his family. He hates his wife and he cannot leave her.

John does not cling to a physical causation, as do those in pain or suffering fatigue, but he does not know he has a depressive illness either. Because he is tortured by his wish for family connection and his hatred of his wife, he is less resistant to counseling. But the counselor may not realize that the underlying cause of his marital problems is not primarily communication difficulties or an immature lack of commitment or his having outgrown or grown apart from his wife, or his recent discovery after twenty years of marriage that she is an "airhead," but the illness of depression. While talking to the counselor about his feelings toward his wife and the importance of maintaining the family may relieve him somewhat and teach him communication skills that are truly useful, the depressive illness must be addressed or the patient and the marriage cannot recover.

John has many of the symptoms of major depressive disorder obscured by the dramatic one that he hates his wife. He suffers from depressed mood, loss of pleasure, sleep disturbance; he has lost weight, has little energy, and feels guilty. John's depression is destroying his family and urgently needs to be treated.

The Job Way

Jeff is a successful lawyer, and has been for twelve years. Married with two kids, he has worked hard for his partnership and house in suburban New York. He needs his large salary, but for the last year he has found the law boring. There seems no point in helping one large corporation get or keep money away from another. Finding the simple winning line in a complicated litigation no longer excites him. He would like to do something that has more social value, like teaching disadvantaged children or helping the sick. But the thought of a second career, especially a low-paying one, seems out of the question. What would happen to his home, and how would he pay the private school tuition?

Joe is an auto mechanic who no longer takes any pleasure in discovering what is wrong with a customer's car and fixing it. Several years ago he switched from a large garage to a much smaller one so that he would have more personal contact with the individual car owner. For a while this seemed to cheer him up, but lately he no longer cares, even when he is complimented on his excellent work. The challenge is gone; the work seems dirty and arduous; and he wishes he could go back to school and become an engineer who designs cars, rather than a grease monkey working on them. But the change seems impossible, and he drags himself along, dreaming on, from day to day.

The lawyer and the auto mechanic just described have been referred to as "burned out," "in midlife crisis," narcissistic, immature, needing to grow up and face adult responsibility, and requiring a spiritual awakening. In fact, these two men are depressed; their depressed mood is expressed in their boredom and hopelessness, their loss of interest and pleasure in their work (not their loved ones), their troubled sleep, their lessened energy, their diminished ability to concentrate, their slowed thoughts and movements on the job. But they do not go to a psychiatrist and say they are depressed. They do not see themselves as depressed, and do not recognize their change in mood, thinking, behavior, and physical capacity as depression. Their spouses, families, friends, physicians, and vocational counselors also do not realize they are ill.

Are You Depressed, or Is This Simply Life?

The abrupt onset of symptoms in each of the four categories of depression (mood, mind, behaviors, and body) makes the diagnosis fairly obvious, if not for the sufferer, then at least for the family, friends, or psychiatrist. When the mood is depressed, the mind disinterested, unable to concentrate, indecisive, filled with self-loathing and suicidal thoughts, when the behavior is constantly restless or completely slowed, when the body is altered by sleep disturbance, appetite or weight change, frequent pain, or loss of sexual interest, then the diagnosis is obvious. But when you are angry, bored, or unhappy, and you think you know the cause (your job, your spouse, your ungrateful children, or whatever else you hold responsible for your hopeless misery), you ought to consider the possibility of major depressive disorder being responsible. When you get the right cause and effective treatment, you will be saved a lot of suffering, not to mention needless divorces and job changes.

A significant percentage of my patients remain uncertain about whether to start antidepressant medication. They explore the deep hurts and abuses of their early childhoods in psychotherapy, or just go out and live life without outside help. Some of them are open to my opinion on the choice of therapy; others are not. Most of you reading this book either are simply curious about antidepressant drugs or are considering taking one. By the time most people pick up a book like this or consult a psychiatrist, they have been in pain for a long time and are unable to get out of it on their own. It is, in my opinion, a sign of health to know when to ask for help. While self-sufficiency is admirable, knowing when to seek assistance is intelligent. Of course, the decision has to do not with logic but with emotion, and many people are opposed to sharing their pain with anyone, even a professional. Progress has been made in the public's acceptance of psychiatric illness, but there's a long way to go, and thus many remain ashamed and unwilling to admit their troubles.

People with major depression benefit from the psychotherapeutic exploration of early childhood deprivations and abuse, but they do not magically recover as a result of this work. In fact, the depression itself operates selectively, causing sufferers to focus on past physical and emotional deprivation and abuse. While the early hurts contribute to the present illness, the current depression blackens the memories and strengthens their effect. Going over these past wrongs, whether real or imagined, does not make the depression go away. Sometimes it even deepens it. This is not a condemnation of the exploration of childhood in psychotherapy, which can be very valuable in terms of identifying the adult's emotional scars and dysfunctional patterns; rather, it is a caution regarding its efficacy in relieving major depressive illness. Most depression experts concur that the psychotherapy of depression must be of a different type from the exploration of childhood.

Should You Try One
of the New Antidepressants?

Because depression can destroy a sufferer's hope for treatment of any kind, and can mire the person down with fatigue
and indecision, and because this disease can also distort
reality so he believes the suffering is deserved and should not
be relieved, and because the illness may worsen gradually
over months so that the individual is unaware that he rarely
speaks, has lost the capacity for spontaneous activity, and no
longer smiles, it is frequently necessary that the opinions of
those who know the person be sought. While the list of
depressive symptoms will aid a patient's self-diagnosis, the
observations of friends, family, and trusted colleagues can
help the individual decide whether to seek treatment. By the
time the observations of those closest might be most valuable,
they may have become angry with the patient, because many
depressed people are very needy. They wear out their spouses
and relatives with their angry, clingy behavior. It is essential
that the depressed person pick someone whose objective
description is not motivated by anger. If this person or several
people all concur that the depressed person seems changed,
down, not his or her normal self, then this is further reason to
consider one of the new antidepressants.

The next two steps involve the family physician, and then the
expert psychiatrist or psychopharmacologist. That is because
many medical diseases mimic psychiatric ones. The opposite is
also true. Thus, psychiatric patients go to medical offices complaining of aches and pains caused by their emotional conditions, while those with unsuspected medical illnesses may be
erroneously referred to psychiatrists. Unfortunately, most primary care physicians have neither the time nor, in many cases,
the knowledge to deal with the complexities of psychiatric illness. It is the expert psychiatrist or psychopharmacologist who
must be consulted for his or her knowledge of both medical
and psychiatric conditions; which are which; how to manage

the two at the same time; and how to factor in the occupation, social, and family aspects of the patient's life.

If you are not sure whether you or a loved one has a major depressive disorder, or wonder if it might be some other form of depression, or suspect there is something wrong but are reluctant to seek help, here are some ways to think about the decision.

You Have Tried to Help Yourself and Failed.

There is a lot of help out there, and some of the people I have seen have tried a fair amount of it, from diet to exercise, vitamins to vacations, workshop weekends to religious retreats, gurus to face-lifts, career change to spouse change, a new hobby, and mind control, and some or all have worked for a little while, and then no longer. Eventually, such attempts at self-help are abandoned because the person becomes discouraged, begins to believe nothing will help, and gives up. If the individual then sinks into the symptoms of depression I have already described, then such a person is a candidate for psychopharmacological evaluation, and perhaps one of the new antidepressants. This decision should not be made in five minutes by matching a list of symptoms to those of major depression, but by a detailed and careful examination.

Psychotherapy Alone Has Failed.

Barbara began therapy when her six-year marriage started to fail. She wanted children and finally decided that Charles, her thirty-six-year-old husband, was more likely to act like a child himself than to father one. After much discussion, they agreed to separate and divorce. She felt she would never marry again, considered having a child anyway, but could not see how she could manage alone on the salary from her job at an insurance company. She found no one to date, withdrew from friends, and derived no pleasure from each day. She lost weight, had no interest in sex, and dragged herself to work. All day she only looked forward to getting home, having several glasses of wine, and watching TV. She had no energy for phone conversations and refused the few offers her friends made, and soon they began to call less and less.

Barbara's therapy did not halt her decline. Rehashing her childhood seemed an academic exercise, and exhortations to make phone calls, see friends, and keep in touch with her family not only did not improve her situation, they made her feel worse. She liked her therapist, found her kind and well-meaning, even competent, but it was clear to Barbara that she was getting worse, not better. Her sister called her one day and recommended that she see a psychiatrist skilled in the administering of antidepressants. At first she snapped at her sister, but slowly she began to wonder if perhaps she was right. She got a referral and decided to see a psychopharmacologist.

Your Temper and Irritability Are Harming You and Your Loved Ones.

Joe and his wife have been married for twenty years. She does everything—taking care of him and the kids, doing the cooking, planning their active social life, and in addition, her earnings amount to half their income. Without her, the phone would not ring, no meals would be cooked, and the children's busy schedules would be in disarray. In spite of all her efforts, Joe criticizes her constantly, shouts at her unmercifully whenever she makes a real or imagined mistake, blames her for any money shortage or problem with the children. His temper has gotten so bad that his wife has begun to speak of it to her minister and to her close friends. Joe's attempts to calm himself with alcohol only make him worse. He is not a nice drunk. One of his wife's friends recommends psychiatric help and she says something to Joe. Naturally, he screams louder.

The new antidepressant drugs calm rages and smooth tempers. These are not official uses of them—they are intended only for major depression—but they are nonetheless widely prescribed for this purpose, and they work effectively. Persuading Joe to go to a psychiatrist will require mobilization of his friends and family, and perhaps assistance from the minister and the family doctor. His wife may even have to threaten to leave. She is determined that he get psychiatric help, because living with him has become a nightmare.

You Have Low Self-Esteem.

The subject of low self-esteem could occupy this whole book, and certainly has in the case of many others. It refers to a chronic low opinion of the self to which the person is so accustomed that he or she does not consider it an illness. People with low self-esteem hide in bad jobs and bad relationships, convinced not only that they deserve no better but that if they were discovered, they would lose the little they have. By hiding in a job, I mean they do their work, take no chances, never complain, and hope the boss will leave them alone. Were they to be found out, they fear they would certainly be fired, since they consider their performance and themselves inadequate. The same is true of their marriage. They allow themselves to be badly treated by their families and friends because they believe themselves inadequate. Such people tend to be poorly paid, to be overlooked for promotion, to feel mistreated by their spouses and children, and to expect no relief. In fact, they have no hope that anything can change for the better.

You Have Chronic Pain.

Your chronic pain may be located in your head (headache, migraine), stomach or bowel, or in your back, and nothing you have done in the past has found its cause or cure. A trial on the new antidepressants may provide the answer to your difficulties.

You Have Insomnia.

Insomnia is a complex and widespread problem that goes beyond the scope of this book. Especially when there is a depressed pattern involving difficulty falling asleep, frequent awakenings, and early-morning awakening, an antidepressant medication may prove very helpful, even in the absence of full depression.

You Have Chronic Fatigue Syndrome.

In the nineteenth century, those who took to their beds in the absence of a clear medical reason were considered neurasthenic. This was sometimes an unfair attribution, because the medical cause existed but remained undetected. Presently, there are a number of people with chronic fatigue syndrome who are not suffering from a viral disorder or an undiscovered medical one, but who do not meet the criteria for major depressive disorder. These patients may respond to an antidepressant medication, and deserve a trial of one.

You Have Bulimia.

Those who are bulimic may respond to an antidepressant. Family studies have revealed a high rate of major affective disorder in the relatives of bulimics. Bulimia refers to recurrent episodes of binge eating followed by a compensatory effort to prevent weight gain, such as by inducing vomiting or taking a laxative. Treatment usually involves a combination of cognitive, behavioral, and drug therapy.

You Have Panic Disorder.

Panic disorder is characterized by sudden attacks of overwhelming fear which are accompanied by a pounding heart and trouble catching one's breath. The person feels dizzy and becomes afraid they are about to die. The first panic attack may occur for no apparent reason, or may follow a serious illness or accident, loss of a loved one, separation from family, childbirth, a thyroid condition, or abuse of a drug like LSD, marijuana, or cocaine. Patients may be convinced they are having a heart attack or losing their sanity. Usually the attacks last no more than twenty minutes. Subsequent attacks occur unexpectedly and fairly often and seem to be associated with deep, rapid breathing. Small doses of the older antidepressants have been very effective in blocking panic attacks, but not the fearful anticipation of them. Low doses of Prozac and Luvox have also been effective. Treatment takes three to ten weeks to work and must be continued for at least six months, but many patients require long-term treatment.

What Are the Types of Mood Disorders?

Major depressive disorder is characterized by one or more major depressive episodes. These episodes, as previously described, consist of at least two weeks of depressed mood or loss of interest plus four of seven other symptoms of depression and no manic or hypomanic episodes. In addition, the depressive moods should not be due to substance abuse, a general medical condition, or schizophrenia.

Dysthymic disorder (dysthymia) refers to a depressed mood over a period of at least two years, accompanied by two or more of the following symptoms: poor appetite (or overeating), insomnia or excessive sleeping, low energy or fatigue, low self-esteem, poor concentration or difficulty making decisions, and feelings of hopelessness. If a person has had a major depressive episode within the past two years, then the diagnosis becomes major depressive episode in partial remission rather than dysthymia. The diagnosis of dysthymia is also not appropriate if the patient has ever been manic or hypomanic or chronically schizophrenic or if the condition is due to substance abuse or a general medical condition. Furthermore, the symptoms must cause significant distress or impairment in social, occupational, or other areas of functioning. Dysthymic disorder can begin in childhood, adolescence, or early adult life, and is chronic in nature.

Dysthymia, also referred to as chronic mild depression, has defied psychiatrists' efforts to define it. In the past, it was called depressive neurosis. The condition lies between major depression and the normal. When an individual has felt sad, hopeless, worried, gloomy, pessimistic, quick to take offense, easily hurt, and discouraged since childhood, she becomes accustomed to it. Depending on her beliefs, she may think life is not easy, rather than that she is ill. When Thomas Hobbes described the life of man in a state of nature as "solitary, poor, nasty, brutish, and short," was he doing so as a philosopher or a dysthymic? Are we to regard the sunny optimist as healthy and the dark pessimist as sick? A patient is not considered dys-thymic if there is a "real" reason for it, such as a general medical condition or schizophrenia, but how about the death of a parent at an early age, or continuous physical or emo-tional abuse? Should we also include poverty, war, imprison-ment, and poor diet as reasons for chronic mild depression coupled with low self-esteem, fatigue, and insomnia? I am afraid that efforts to place dysthymia in the biological camp and outside the psychological one—in the area of the chemi-cal and out of the experiential—are unconvincing to me. Yet there is no question that antidepressants can sometimes treat this condition more effectively than psychotherapy. Just because a drug is effective in treating a psychiatric condition does not make its etiology hereditary or chemical. We are all ultimately composed of chemicals. If a lion were to walk into my office, the chemistry of my body and that of my patient would immediately change radically. If you did not know about the lion, but only measured the elements of the blood, you might think a chemical imbalance existed, when, in fact, the cause was fear of the lion.

Major Depressive Disorder: Will You Get Sick Again?

In over half the cases, major depressive disorder is a recurring illness. This is something that those who are not expert in the study and treatment of depression may forget. That is why it is necessary to obtain a careful history of the patient's life. What was he like before he became depressed? Was he optimistic, productive, functioning well in work and outside, or was he dysthymic, gloomy, withdrawn, and chronically depressed? Is this the first or one of several episodes, and is there any pattern to what brings them on? One first-year graduate student came to my office because he found it very difficult to go to class and do his work. He wondered if perhaps he just did not want to become an economist and perhaps should have gotten a job after college and not sought a graduate degree. It was tempting to enter fully into a discussion with him of the pros and cons of economics, the dismal science, and of job prospects post-Ph.D., which also seemed dismal. But instead of prematurely beginning psychotherapy, I did as I usually do and took a careful history. His first year in college had also been very shaky. In fact, he had dropped out, gotten a job, and gone back to school, enrolling at an institution nearer to his close family. He went home each weekend, his laundry in tow, for a good meal and long talks with his mother. His first year of high school was also stressful, as he tried to fit in with a new group of classmates. He wondered if the others accepted him, and he felt especially awkward with girls. His grades initially suffered, but he was able to pull them up. It became clear that he was suffering his third depression, each brought on by the stress associated with transferring to a new school and separation from his close-knit family. The problem was not in economic graduate school, it was in him. First his mood needed to be improved, and then he could decide whether to continue. It was clear he had a mild form of a major depressive disorder: he took less interest and pleasure in his studies, had trouble sleeping, appeared tense and agitated, lacked energy, was unable to concentrate on his work, and had little hope for the future. Six weeks later, on 20 mg of Paxil daily, he was attending classes with interest and beginning to make friends. He continued to wonder if he should content himself with an M.A. in economics and then go to work, or stay on for a Ph.D. All his problems, including his excessive dependence on his family, had not been solved by Paxil, but he now had the energy to face them.

The course of major depressive disorder varies: there are otherwise healthy individuals who have a single episode and those who have many episodes; there are those who are asymptomatic between attacks and others who only partially recover, as well as some who never do. About 20 percent of major depression sufferers become chronic and remain partly or completely incapacitated by the disease. It is the physician's job to study the pattern of the illness and to vigorously treat it in order to prevent, or at least minimize, incapacity. Prompt, vigorous dosage of the proper antidepressant alone, or in combination with another medication, plus suitable psychotherapy, can rehabilitate the patient and allow him to lead a full, productive life.

Depression and Mania

Now called bipolar disorder, manic-depressive illness can severely disrupt a person's life. I will discuss the relationship between major depression and bipolar disorder, but a full description of this serious illness would require an additional volume. Nonetheless, it is necessary to pay it some attention because some major depressives evolve into bipolars, and because all antidepressant medications carry the potential for converting depression into mania.

Manic Episode

A manic episode is characterized by a persistent elevated or irritable mood lasting more than one week and accompanied by inflated self-esteem, decreased need for sleep, rapid speech, distractibility, racing thoughts, and participation in many sexual and occupational activities. Manic individuals embark on an array of activities, often completing none. They are restless and get involved in buying sprees, imprudent business ventures, and unusual sexual activities, even with strangers. The disturbance is severe enough that the patient requires protection from the negative consequences of his poor business, sexual, illegal, or assaultive behavior. The symptoms of a manic episode may be caused by antidepressant medication, shock therapy, or drugs like corticosteroids. When drug-caused, the manic episode is not diagnosed as Bipolar I Disorder (also known as manic depression), but as Substance-Induced Mood Disorder with Manic Features. Patients during a manic episode usually do not recognize that something is wrong and consequently resist treatment. The patient may dress bizarrely, travel impulsively, become sexually aggressive, and engage in giving unsolicited advice to strangers. Ethical concerns may be disregarded and the patient may become assaultive. His or her poor judgment and excessive activity can lead to brushes with the law or large monetary losses. The patient's mood may rapidly shift to anger or depression. The patient may use large amounts of drugs or alcohol. Depressive symptoms are usually brief, lasting minutes or hours. If manic and depressive symptoms are significantly present every day for a week, the condition is considered Bipolar I, mixed type.

The first manic episode usually occurs between the ages of twenty and twenty-five, and begins suddenly with a rapid increase over a few days. Mania lasts several weeks or months, and the episodes are shorter than those of major depression. A major depressive episode often immediately precedes or follows a manic one.

Hypomanic Episode

A hypomanic episode is one in which an elevated, expansive, or irritable mood lasts at least four days and is accompanied by any three of the following: inflated self-esteem, grandiosity, little need for sleep, rapid speech, racing thoughts, distractibility, excessive involvement in activities and pleasures. Whereas manic episodes may be accompanied by delusions and hallucinations, hypomanic ones are not. To be considered hypomanic, the mood must be clearly different from the person's usual one, but not severe enough to completely disrupt work or social activities or require hospitalization. When there is a known cause for the manic or hypomanic episode, such as hyperthyroidism or an antidepressant medication, the patient is considered not to be bipolar, but to have manic features due to the medical condition or drug.

The hypomanic's mood is cheerful and unusually high, but may switch to irritability, and his or her speech may be filled with jokes and puns.

Bipolar I Disorder

To be considered Bipolar I (formerly manic-depressive), a patient must have had at least one manic episode. About 15 percent of major depressives will become Bipolar I patients. Unlike major depressive disorder, which is more common in women, Bipolar I Disorder affects men and women equally. Ninety percent of those having a single manic episode have subsequent ones, and about two thirds of manic episodes occur just before or after a major depressive one. Untreated, patients have four episodes in ten years on average, and the interval decreases as the patient gets older. About 10 percent of Bipolar I patients have four episodes of mood disorder (major depressive, manic, mixed, or hypomanic) per year, and these are called rapid cyclers. Most Bipolar I patients are normal between episodes, but about 20 percent are not.

While studies show evidence of genetic influence in Bipolar I Disorder, it should be remembered that the large majority of individuals with Bipolar I close relatives do not become Bipolar I themselves. Bipolar disorders constitute 20 percent of all major mood disorders. Most bipolar disorders are treated with either lithium, Depakote (valproic acid), Tegretol, an antipsychotic (e.g., Haldol) or antianxiety drug (e.g., Klonopin) for the manic phase, and an antidepressant for the depressed phase.

Bipolar II Disorder

People who suffer hypomanic and major depressive episodes but may only remember and be troubled by their downs, and not by their highs, have Bipolar II Disorder. It is often their friends and relatives who identify the periods of elevated or irritable mood, rapid speech, lack of sleep, distractibility, buying sprees, sexual indiscretions, and foolish investments. The frequency of Bipolar II episodes is the same as that of Bipolar I.

It is important to distinguish bipolar from unipolar (episodes of depression only, no mania or hypomania) because it influences which drugs a patient should be given. The unsuspected Bipolar II can be tipped over into mania or hypomania by an antidepressant drug. Diagnosis is not merely an exercise in naming; it involves an assessment as to what is likely to happen in the future and how the patient should be treated.

Cyclothymic Disorder

An individual is considered cyclothymic if he has chronic mood swings that are not severe enough to constitute major depression or full mania. The mood swings must interfere with important parts of the patient's life, making him moody and unpredictable. Cyclothymic disorder usually begins in adolescence, and may go on to become Bipolar I or II Disorder.

Mild hypomania and mild depression are hard to distinguish from normal behavior. Whether an individual is merely moody or cyclothymic can be hard to decide, but the distinction is clearer if an attempt is made to judge whether the episode represents a change "uncharacteristic of the person when not symptomatic" (*Diagnostic and Statistical Manual*, 4th ed., 1994). Lithium and other mood-stabilizing drugs are as effective in cyclothymics as they are in bipolar patients. The cyclothymic patients who find their periods of hypomania productive and their depressions tolerable do not need mood-stabilizing medications.

What Causes Depression?

In *The American Psychiatric Press Textbook of Psychiatry* (2d ed., 1994), the causes of depression are listed under three main headings—biological, psychological, and genetic—and under each of these are a half dozen or more models and theories. This textbook begins its discussion of the causes of major depressive disorder and bipolar disorder by saying they are "unknown" and that "a thoroughly satisfying explanation for the effectiveness of treatments is lacking." In clinical practice, I primarily find patients who fit each of the main textbook headings, and believe that the cause is biological, psychological, or hereditary. I believe that many of these people are correct in their estimate of the cause of their own depression. One woman insisted her depression was caused by the fact that she no longer loved her husband but could not divorce him because of the children. She refused to take an antidepressant drug. A salesman saw no reason to talk about his problems. He had heard that Prozac was very effective and wanted to try it. Then he would have renewed confidence and be able to go out on sales calls. The mother believed her depression to be psychologically caused, and the salesman biologically. Since there is an interplay between the inner biological state and the world outside, it makes sense that for one person, life events can be the main source of depression, and for another, bodily chemistry.

The genetic link for depression is stronger for people with bipolar disorder than for those with unipolar (major depression only) disorder. The incidence of mood disorder in relatives of unipolar patients is twice the rate in relatives of people without mood disorder, which translates to 10 percent versus 5 percent. This is a significant, but not overwhelming, association, which means that the relatives of unipolar patients are far from certain to get the disease. The hereditary line in bipolar disorder is much stronger, with about 25 percent of the relatives of a bipolar patient being either bipolar or unipolar.

The Biochemical (Neurotransmitter) Theory

Neurotransmitters are chemical substances that cross the gap from one nerve cell to the next (called the synapse) in order to stimulate or inhibit that cell. Originally, it was thought that too much of the neurotransmitters norepinephrine and serotonin caused mania, and too little caused depression. But because it could not be consistently shown that depressives had too little serotonin and norepinephrine, and because there was a several-week lag between the time these neurotransmitters were increased by antidepressant drugs and the first signs of clinical improvement, other explanations became necessary. Research attention has shifted from the synapse to the interior of the nerve cell to account for the time lag.

Other theories accounting for depression include thyroid abnormalities, with low thyroid activity (hypothyroid) accounting for depression and an overactive thyroid (hyperthyroid) accounting for mania. Those depressives who do not get better on antidepressants may improve when thyroid medication is added.

Psychological Theories

Psychoanalytic theories of depression emphasize the loss of love or status by a person made excessively vulnerable by extraordinary frustrations (or dissatisfactions) in childhood. Susceptible individuals made overly dependent because of early trauma react to a loss with the feeling that all is gone and the world is now empty. Their self-esteem severely diminished, they feel they are no good and no one loves them. Early deprivations made these people needy and angry and predispose them to depression. In psychoanalytic theory, frustration makes the vulnerable angry and the anger turns inward, causing depression.

Dr. Aaron Beck is a psychiatrist who devised the theory of cognitive behavior. Beck's theory is that depression (and other psychological problems) are caused by the way one thinks. Beck believes that depression is caused by negative views of the self, the environment, and the future which have been learned during childhood and adolescence. Dr. Beck has devised an effective psychotherapy of depression which teaches how to identify negative thinking patterns and how to reverse them.

The relationship of depression to life events can be difficult to establish. For example, did the patient become depressed because she was divorced, or was she divorced because she was depressed? Studies of the effect of a parent's death in early childhood as a cause of later depression show this to be an important event, but not as powerful as some psychoanalysts suggest. Stresses such as the death of, separation from, or strife with important people in the patient's life or failures and disappointments are more important in first episodes of depression than in later ones. The later episodes of depression are more easily elicited by weaker and weaker stresses once the initial pattern has been set, until it may become difficult to identify any trauma causing a relapse.

A Combination Theory of the Cause of Depression

Two veterans of the horrors of war come home having had almost identical experiences. One is hospitalized with post-traumatic stress disorder and relives his terror in flashbacks, while the other prospers in his new job. Why the difference? There is an interaction of life events and the makeup of the person to whom they happen. This makeup consists of heredity and environment, both of which shape the individual who experiences the trauma. That is why the early death of a parent does not inevitably lead to depression. It depends on the child's heredity, life experiences prior to the death, and what happens afterward. This after-experience can be seen in the effect of divorce on children. It has been shown that if both parents maintain positive contact with the child afterward, the damage of divorce is minimized.

There are more than a dozen different types of depression. In addition, the fate of patients within a depressive category varies dramatically. This is well known in physical medicine, where one victim may die of a heart attack, and another live thirty years longer, where one arthritic person may complain of aches and pains, and another cannot walk. Similarly, one patient may become depressed after being fired from a job, but will snap back, while another will take to her bed for a year. Studies of abortion show that while most women are upset by it, only those with a tendency to succumb to stress become emotionally ill. Why some are vulnerable to stress and others possess the capacity for resilience is not understood. Insofar as a person's vulnerabilities are unique to the individual, each person must study his or her own, sometimes with the aid of a psychiatrist or psychotherapist, in order to learn to resist them better and bounce back faster.

It remains hard to explain why depressions often occur spontaneously and then disappear completely after about six months. If there is a biochemical abnormality, then why does it come and go? If it has something to do with serotonin, then why would the serotonin system go out of balance and then back in balance? Much progress has been made in the understanding of this terrible affliction, but the puzzle remains.

What Are Antidepressants?

Antidepressants are drugs that are used to treat depression. They are often prescribed by general practitioners, psychiatrists, and by psychopharmacologists; the latter are medical psychiatrists who specialize in the study of the effects on behavior of drugs, as well as naturally occurring substances within the body, such as serotonin. Psychopharmacologists are keenly interested in the design and development of safer and more effective antidepressants. It is through their cooperation with research scientists at drug companies that the new, improved antidepressants were, and continue to be, developed.

Before these specialists existed, drug discovery depended entirely on serendipity. For example, the antituberculosis agent Iproniazid produced unexpected mood elevation in tuberculosis patients. Following up on this finding in 1957, scientists discovered that this drug did indeed have antidepressant efficacy in psychiatric patients. Thus, the first monoamine oxidase inhibitor was introduced to psychiatry. In the early 1950s, the Swiss psychiatrist Roland Kuhn investigated several agents chemically similar to Thorazine, a drug that had just been discovered to be effective in the treatment of schizophrenia. He was looking for a treatment for depression, and after treating his first three cases in 1956, he discovered the first tricyclic antidepressant, imipramine (Tofranil), a close chemical cousin of Thorazine. John Cade, an unknown Australian psychiatrist who had no research training, was investigating the effect produced by injecting the urine of manic patients into guinea pigs. He chose to dissolve the urine's uric acid in water by combining it with lithium, the acid's most soluble salt. When injected into guinea pigs, lithium made the urine less toxic, so he became interested in studying lithium itself. He found that lithium carbonate injected into guinea pigs made them lethargic. Next, he tried lithium in ten manic patients in 1948 and found their excitement to be controlled.

In the last twenty years, antidepressants have begun to be designed based on neuroscience, rather than discovered by chance. Thus, cleaner drugs affecting only serotonin have been developed, producing many fewer side effects than the older antidepressants, which affected a variety of neurotransmitters, some of which were irrelevant to their clinical effect. Progress in designing new antidepressants is slow, because the brain contains about 10 billion cells, and more than fifty known neurotransmitters along with many unknown others, which influence many targets and produce varying effects on cell genes. In spite of this extraordinary complexity, progress is being made. Once the drug is designed, the gradual process of careful testing begins. It was fifteen years from the development of Prozac in 1972 by the scientists of Eli Lilly to its release by the U.S. Food and Drug Administration for public use in 1987.

In order for the FDA to allow the release of a new antidepressant, it must be safe and effective. Safety applies not only to the four to six weeks of a controlled clinical trial but to the long term. About 2,500 patients are given the investigational new agent and assessed for safety, but only several hundred of them are observed for more than a few months. The antidepressants nomifensine, bupropion (Wellbutrin), and zimelidine have been withdrawn from the U.S. market, although bupropion was rereleased with new prescribing instructions. The safety of a drug must be carefully monitored after its release, not just before.

The effectiveness of any antidepressant is a complicated subject. The four- to six-week controlled trial comparing the active agent usually only to a placebo, but sometimes to another proven antidepressant, is used to show that the new drug is statistically superior to the placebo. But this leaves two very important issues unaddressed. The first is an acute short-term one: that the difference between the drug and the placebo may be mathematically and statistically significant, but unimpressive clinically. That is, the patient may feel somewhat better—better than if he or she were on a sugar pill—but not completely well. Many psychopharmacologists have recommended that these trials be longer than the four to six weeks required by law so that the patients will have enough time to improve clinically, not just statistically. The second effectiveness issue is the long-term one. Drug side effects that a patient notices or is willing to tolerate during acute deep depression may become intolerable in the long term. For example, the patient may not care about medication interfering with sexual functioning while deeply depressed, but may, once he or she is feeling better, stop taking the drug for this reason. A drug that produces side effects of sufficient magnitude that patients stop taking it obviously loses its value. Since depression recurs in more than 50 percent of patients, the effectiveness of an antidepressant is very much influenced by a patient's willingness to continue to remain on it.

What Is Improvement?

Full recovery may be used in reference to a person being totally asymptomatic, whereas *partial recovery* means that some symptoms remain, but not enough for the depression to be considered major. A *relapse* is defined as a return of symptoms during an ongoing treated episode. This happens when drug therapy is stopped too soon. *Recurrence* describes a new episode of major depression following the cure of a previous one. The importance of these distinctions, especially between relapse and recurrence, lies in deciding whether an acute episode has been treated long enough or whether the patient should be maintained on an antidepressant to prevent recurrence of new episodes.

Mood disorders have traditionally been thought to be episodic, with a good prognosis. This long-held view has been modified, however, by careful research. While the general outcome remains positive, 20 percent of major depressives are now believed to become chronic, 30 percent are unresponsive to antidepressant medication, and as many as 40-plus percent do not get well or are intolerant to the first drug tried. Half of these will respond to a second drug, and still more to innovative drug combinations.

While a total cure is the goal of every antidepressant drug treatment, it must be remembered that residual symptoms are all too common; they also imply a higher risk of relapse and prevent the depressed person from full participation in work and at home.

Three of the main rating scales used in evaluating new drugs in depression are the Hamilton, the global, and the Zung self-rating scales. The Hamilton is used in every study of a new antidepressant drug. It contains the following 17 items and rates each on a 3- or a 5-point severity scale.

1. depressed mood
2. guilt
3. suicide
4. initial insomnia (difficulty falling asleep)
5. middle sleep insomnia (waking up in the middle of the night)

6. delayed insomnia (waking up too early and being unable to go back to sleep)
7. work and interests
8. retardation
9. agitation
10. anxiety—psychic (fearful thoughts, worry, tension, irritability, feeling jumpy)
11. anxiety—somatic (fast pulse, abdominal distress, frequent urination)
12. somatic symptoms—gastrointestinal (loss of appetite)
13. somatic symptoms—general (fatigue, muscle aches)
14. genital symptoms (loss of libido)
15. hypochondriasis
16. loss of insight
17. loss of weight

A total score indicates the number of symptoms and their severity. Severe depression is indicated by a score over 28, moderate depression between 14 and 28. Patients do not feel truly well until the score is under 6. In the four-week studies required by the FDA before antidepressants can be released, scores must fall by 50 percent for a drug to be considered effective. Typically, a drop from a Hamilton average of 24 to 12 occurs while the placebo fall is statistically significantly less, perhaps 24 to 15. At a Hamilton score of 12, the patient continues to feel badly. For this reason, many psychopharmacologists recommend that the trials be extended until the patients are completely recovered.

The Zung scale consists of a list of depressive symptoms which is self-administered by the patient and scored by the doctor. The global scale is the doctor's overall impression of the severity of the patient's condition.

Antidepressant Drugs Available in the United States

Generic Name   Brand Name

Monoamine Oxidase Inhibitors
phenelzine   Nardil
tranylcypromine   Parnate

Heterocyclic Antidepressants
imipramine   Tofranil, etc.
amitriptyline   Elavil, etc.
trimipramine   Surmontil
doxepin   Sinequan, etc.
amoxapine   Asendin
clomipramine   Anafranil
desipramine   Norpramin, etc.
nortriptyline   Aventyl, Pamelor
protriptyline   Vivactil
maprotiline   Ludiomil

Selective Serotonin Reuptake Inhibitors
fluoxetine   Prozac
sertraline   Zoloft
paroxetine   Paxil
fluvoxamine   Luvox

Other Antidepressants (Unclassified)
bupropion   Wellbutrin
trazodone   Desyrel, etc.
nefazodone   Serzone
venlafaxine   Effexor
mirtazapine   Remeron

Monoamine Oxidase Inhibitors (MAOIs)

Monoamine oxidase inhibitors (MAOIs) are drugs that
inhibit the enzyme monoamine oxidase from breaking down

the neurotransmitters norepinephrine, serotonin, and dopamine and therefore cause the amount of each of them to rise. Nardil and Parnate are MAOIs that are effective in the treatment of major depression, especially so in atypical depression and also in bipolar depression. The main side effects of these drugs are sedation, dizziness, rapid heartbeat, insomnia, sexual dysfunction, constipation, and agitation. Their main disadvantage is the sudden severe elevation of blood pressure following intake of certain foods and medications. Patients cannot eat aged meats and cheeses and cannot take certain over-the-counter cold medications. The hypertension that may be induced can lead to headache, vomiting, palpitations, and occasionally to a stroke. Because of these side effects, MAOIs are typically not the first drugs used to treat depression. New, safer MAOIs are under investigation but so far have not been released.

Heterocyclic Antidepressants

Heterocyclic antidepressants (which include most tricyclics) were the most commonly used antidepressants for thirty years, given to millions of patients with excellent results. In fact, none of the new antidepressants are more effective than the 70 percent response rate achieved by these older agents. The selective serotonin reuptake inhibitors (SSRIs) like Prozac were developed because Elavil and Tofranil blocked serotonin reuptake, as well as that of norepinephrine, and it was hoped that the SSRIs would be as effective, yet less toxic. The tricyclic antidepressants (the term *tricyclic* refers to the chemical structure of drugs such as Elavil and Tofranil) have been used in many conditions other than depression. These include panic attacks, migraine, chronic pain, bed-wetting, and bulimia. In addition, the older drugs were tested on hospitalized major depressives whereas the new SSRIs have mainly been researched in outpatients. Originally, it was believed that the more toxic tricyclic antidepressants might be more effective in the treatment of serious depressions requiring hospitalization. Their broad spectrum of action, affecting both norepinephrine and serotonin along with various other neurotransmitters responsible for their troublesome side effects, caused some to speculate that the inpatient and outpatient populations on whom the tricyclic and SSRI drug studies had been done were not comparable. Many wondered whether the Elavil- and Tofranil-like drugs might remain the drugs of choice for hospitalized depressives. This seems not to be the case, and many new studies have found the SSRIs to be equally effective in the treatment of severe depression.

It is not their effectiveness but the problems (discussed in the following section) associated with the older antidepressants that have caused their usage to decline.

Side Effects of Tricyclic Antidepressants

Heart and Circulatory

The tricyclics make the pulse speed up by 20 or more beats per minute. This can be frightening or annoying to people with healthy hearts and dangerous to those with a weakened cardiac status. The older antidepressants may disrupt the orderly beat of the heart, either by delaying electrical conduction within cardiac muscle, which can be seen on an electrocardiogram, or on rare occasions causing complete disorder and sudden death. The danger of sudden death is of particular concern in patients with serious heart disease and in children who are being treated with these agents in order to prevent bed-wetting. These drugs also may lower the blood pressure, especially in the elderly, who, when standing up after getting out of bed in the morning, may feel dizzy or light-headed, and sometimes may fall and be injured. The tricyclics have been used safely for years, but now are avoided in favor of the newer antidepressants, especially in cardiac patients. When they must be used, the doctor should take a careful cardiac history, check the blood pressure and pulse, and evaluate the effects of other medical drugs being simultaneously taken; an electrocardiogram is advisable in older people before the tricyclic is prescribed. Follow-up cardiograms are necessary once maximum dosage has been established.

Visual

There are three main visual effects of the tricyclics. Some of the older drugs are worse than others on the eye. These drugs dry the eye and may be hazardous to contact-lens wearers. Artificial-tear preparations may help, but if the problem is severe, use of the drug may have to be stopped. Blurred vision is a second problem, which disturbs the individual's ability to read, especially early on in the treatment. Often this problem disappears after a week or two. The third problem can be avoided by a visit to the ophthalmologist to determine whether the patient has previously unsuspected narrow-angle glaucoma, in which case the older antidepressants pose a serious threat to eyesight and should not be used at all.

Gastrointestinal and Urinary

The older antidepressants are "dirty" drugs, meaning that they affect parts of the body not relevant to their therapeutic action. The same mechanism that dries the eyes also dries the mouth and slows the bowel and the flow of urine. Dry mouth occurs in some depressives not on medication and is worsened by tricyclics, while others experience this annoyance for the first time because of the drug. The effect may be reduced by sugarless lozenges or artificial saliva and often goes away by itself after several weeks, once the individual gets used to the drug. Sometimes dry mouth leads to tooth decay.

Constipation can be a symptom of depression and a side effect of the tricyclics. It can be mild and dealt with by dosage adjustment, fluid intake, or mild laxatives, but on rare occasions it can be severe, especially in older or medically vulnerable patients.

A slow urinary flow, especially in men with enlarged prostates, can be anything from an annoyance to an emergency when complete retention results.

When they are mild, the gastrointestinal and urinary problems are usually waited out in the hope that they will subside as the individual adjusts to the drug. If this does not happen, the dose may be reduced, or alternate antidepressants prescribed. Sometimes a drug such as bethanechol chloride (Urecholine) is successfully added to combat dry mouth, constipation, and urinary difficulties.

Weight Gain

Many patients who have been brought out of deep despair by the tricyclic antidepressants have stopped taking them because of a new misery—the effect on their weight. Some have gained as much as thirty pounds and risked falling back into depression rather than expand further. The reason for this added poundage is not entirely understood. It is not merely the return of pounds previously lost due to depression, nor is it due to swelling up because of water retention. Some investigators have described a carbohydrate craving stimulated by the medicine as well as a slowing of metabolism, but it is not known why this occurs. Some trycyclics such as desipramine and protriptyline seem to cause less weight gain and the Prozac-like SSRI drugs bupropion and nefazodone rarely cause weight gain, another reason why they are desirable.

Sexual Dysfunction

It is necessary to distinguish between those side effects caused by the medication and those caused by the illness itself. Loss of interest in sex is commonly experienced by depressed people who are not on medication. Before any antidepressant is prescribed this pattern must be carefully noted in order to evaluate any change. A person with a painful major depression may complain of many other, more troubling symptoms than loss of sex drive, which may not be mentioned at all. The thorough doctor will ask about sexual desire before prescribing an antidepressant. Then it is possible to differentiate between what is drug-induced and what is a component of the depression which has not yet been successfully treated. A person with major depression who feels better because of medication may begin to complain of loss of sex drive because preoccupation with suicide and the inability to work or care for the family present less of a problem. The remaining sexual difficulty can be caused by depression, prior inhibitions, relationship difficulties, or drugs. A careful evaluation before the drug treatment is started will help immeasurably in deciding the true cause.

Once the individual has fully improved, and it is determined that the tricyclic is to blame for impotence, lack of orgasm, loss of sexual interest, or inability to ejaculate, a decrease in tricyclic dosage may help without causing the person to relapse. If this fails, the antidepressant can be replaced by another one, or other drugs may be given to overcome the problem. Two antidepressants that may be particularly helpful are Wellbutrin and Serzone, and possibly Remeron. Medications that can supplement the original antidepressant to overcome the drug-induced sexual difficulty are bethanechol or the antiserotonin drug cyproheptadine (taken an hour before intercourse to promote orgasm) or yohimbine (to overcome impotence). These three drugs are sometimes helpful but do not always provide the solution.

Suicide Potential

Major depressive disorder and bipolar disorder are serious illnesses with a fatality rate by suicide as high as 15 percent. Experts disagree regarding whether ideas of suicide are

increased or stopped by the old or new antidepressants. However, there is no question that tricyclics are the leading cause
of death by overdose in the United States. It takes only about
a week's supply of a full therapeutic dose of Tofranil or Elavil
for a patient to commit suicide. This sobering fact caused
many family physicians to prescribe very low doses out of fear
that patients would overdose. Thus, many depressives were
inadequately treated by minuscule amounts of medication
that in adequate dosage would have made them well. One
great advantage of the new antidepressants is their much
lower lethality. The tricyclics were found by one reviewer to
be more than five times as likely to cause death by overdose
than Prozac.

Similarities and Differences Among
the New and Old Antidepressants

There is no difference in the cure rate among the twenty
antidepressant drugs now available, with the possible excep-
tion of the monoamine oxidase inhibitors Nardil and Parnate. If the eighteen other drugs are all equally effective in
the approximately 70 percent of patients whose conditions
they improve, then why were some experts reluctant to try the
new ones? Many psychiatrists were at first a little slow in trying
new agents that appeared safe but whose long-term toxicity
was unknown. This attitude is not merely conservatism for its
own sake. The long-term danger of the antipsychotic drug
Thorazine was unknown until seven years after it was released.
Abnormal movements of the face and tongue were noticed in
patients who had been on the drug for more than six months,
and as many as 20 percent of chronic hospitalized patients
suffered this side effect. Worse still, it did not always go away
when use of the drug was stopped, and sometimes it became
worse. Although the initial report of tardive dyskinesia was
published in 1959, seven years after the drug began to be prescribed, it was not until about five years later that the full

extent of the problem became known. It was not uncommon in the 1950s and 1960s for Thorazine and its cousins (e.g., Stelazine) to be given in low doses to people who were not schizophrenic but merely nervous or unable to sleep. Physicians had no idea they were exposing people to the danger of developing these abnormal, permanent facial tics. Of course, a dozen years later, this became widely known, and the practice was stopped. I have spent all this time on Thorazine's late-occurring, unsuspected side effect to remind you that new drugs are not entirely without risk. And the problem with new drugs applies to the antidepressants. Nomifensine, a new antidepressant, was approved by the Food and Drug Administration in 1985 (only two years before Prozac) and then abruptly taken off the market because it attacked and destroyed red blood cells, causing severe anemia. Zimelidine, the first selective serotonin reuptake inhibitor (SSRI), was withdrawn in 1982 because in a small number of cases it caused sudden disease of the nerves leading to muscular weakness and paralysis. Fortunately, this does not seem to be a problem with the others SSRIs—Prozac, Paxil, Zoloft, or Luvox. Finally, Wellbutrin was released by the FDA, then withdrawn because it was associated with a higher incidence of seizures than other antidepressants, and finally rereleased with more stringent dosage guidelines, which seems to have solved the problem. I cite all these mishaps not to excessively frighten you regarding new drugs but to underline the point that we do not know all there is to know about a drug when it is released, and if there are older, equally effective, safe ones, then continuing to use these rather than new ones with unknown dangers makes some sense.

The 70 Percent Cure Rate

Seventy percent of all people taking antidepressants report an improvement, meaning that there is at least a 50 percent reduction in their symptoms. This is in comparison with

40 percent of people taking a placebo, whose symptoms of depression are also relieved. All the antidepressant drugs, new and old, achieve the 70 percent figure. What is not known is whether the various drugs improve the same 70 percent. The clinical suspicion is that different drugs help different patients, but doctors are unable to predict which individual depressed patient will be helped by a certain drug. It was initially thought that since the older antidepressants had been researched in sicker inpatients and the newer ones in less ill outpatients, each type would be most effective in the groups upon which they were tried. While this matter is being intensively researched, it appears that the new antidepressants are as effective in sicker inpatients as the older drugs are.

It is my belief that the new antidepressants do substantially better than the old ones in outpatient depressives. The reason for this is partly that they are better drugs, but mainly that they are being used better. A doctor does not have to be an expert psychopharmacologist to use Prozac better than he used Elavil. Often when he prescribed Elavil he was afraid the patient would overdose, so very small doses were given in case the person took all of them at once. Since the typical family doctor did not see the depressed individual very often, he or she was in no position to trust the patient with a large supply of Elavil. The family doctor typically prescribed too little of the drug, and the patient did not recover. In the relatively rare case where the dosage was adequate, the general practitioner did not see the patient often enough to cope with the side effects, and the patient was likely to stop taking the medication. Only the psychiatrist or psychopharmacologist, who saw the patient more frequently, could encourage the acceptance of dry mouth, dizziness, blurred vision, constipation, and other unpleasant side effects while the dose was being raised to a point where it would be effective. The older antidepressants had dose ranges from one to twelve tablets and required careful increases, from a modest beginning to all twelve tablets in cases where the full amount was required.

This rarely happened. Either the patient received too little of the drug or stopped taking the drug because of a side effect. In either case, he or she did not get better.

With at least half of the new antidepressants, patients require only one tablet a day. The family doctor does not have to carefully raise the dose until an effective level is reached. The drugs have a fairly low lethal potential so that the physician does not fear giving a month's supply at a time. Remember that one week's supply of Elavil could kill a patient.

Finally, the new antidepressants do not make patients faint or cause severe constipation, hand tremors, dry mouth, weight gain, or blurred vision. Because they are tolerated much better, patients do not stop taking them as often before they are successful at reducing symptoms. More patients are completing a full dose for an adequate period of time, are not discontinuing use of the drug against the doctor's advice, and are benefiting. The new drugs are thus doing a substantially better job in outpatient depressives, the majority of whom are being treated not by expert psychopharmacologists but by family doctors. The reason the new antidepressants have made such an impression is that they are easy to prescribe, are safe, can be given in full dose, and produce few side effects.

Remaining Problems

In spite of the great advance in the drug treatment of depression, three serious problems remain. These are the problems of lag time, treatment failures, and side effects.

Lag Time

If a person is severely depressed, preoccupied with suicide, unable to get out of bed, and experiencing difficulty at work or in caring for his or her family, there is a need for the individual to respond to treatment immediately, not after a week, a month, or half a year. In fact, a two-year follow-up study of 101 patients by Dr. Martin Keller et al. found that only 50 percent of these severely depressed people had recovered after one year. Patients with less severe symptoms have a better chance of recovery. The weeks or months of illness take a serious toll on marriage, work, family, and friendships, and increase the danger of suicide. Quick-acting antidepressant drugs must be found, but so far, in spite of claims by some company advertisements, no one medication has been proven to act faster than any other. Nonetheless, the situation is not all that bleak. Antidepressants markedly improve the condition of many patients within several days to a week, and double their chances for recovery within a month. They are among the most effective drugs, both in psychiatry and in all of medicine.

Treatment Failures

Without getting too technical, I must emphasize that there is a big difference between response and cure. A person who responds to a drug may be better able to function but may still suffer some symptoms. Someone who is cured is completely restored to health. While a degree of relief from symptoms is very important, the patient's overall ability to function may remain seriously impaired. It is necessary for the depressed patient to receive an adequate dose for a long enough period before being counted a treatment failure. Too often patients referred to university psychiatric facilities as drug-unresponsive have received inadequate dosages or the wrong medication. When treated properly, they then improve. Proper dosage is not a single standard, but varies from one person to another.

It has been estimated that 40 percent of those who have tried an antidepressant cannot tolerate the side effects or do not respond to the first drug with which they are treated. Of these, an additional 50 percent respond to a second antidepressant, especially if it is of a different type. Thus, someone who fails on an SSRI (like Prozac) might respond to

Wellbutrin. This leaves 20 percent who fail to respond to the second drug. These people are given one of several drugs in addition to the second antidepressant, such as thyroid, lithium, a tricyclic (if the SSRI failed), buspirone, trazodone, Ritalin, or estrogen in women. Many of these combinations seem to work. There is little research evidence to support this, however. Rather, the practice has clinical, anecdotal support. Controlled studies are necessary to establish that the observed improvement is due to the active drugs and not to the passage of time or the placebo effect of changing medicines. With these added drug treatments, over 90 percent eventually respond—a very fine result—but unfortunately, 5 or 10 percent do not.

Side Effects

The trouble with the older antidepressants was that many people could not tolerate them at all, or were unable to accept high enough doses to get the full benefit. As a result, many stopped taking them, or were maintained on such low amounts that they received little help. The physician who used them properly was in the position of encouraging patients to suffer more discomfort on the drug than their depression had made them suffer in the first place, until one to three weeks had elapsed and they began to feel better. By this time, the side effects often seemed to subside as the person became used to the medicine and felt better.

The new antidepressants are much better tolerated and represent a great advance. Nonetheless, about 15 to 20 percent of people who take them cannot tolerate the abdominal distress or "drugged" feeling, or other side effects, and must stop taking the medication. An equal number do not improve, so that the figure of about 40 or more percent who fail to improve on their first antidepressant remains. This situation is not unique to psychiatry. Many medical patients on blood pressure medication either cannot tolerate or fail to respond to the first drug tried. People who are depressed are in pain, and their ability to function is often hampered. It would be best if the doctor knew which type of depressed patient would respond to which drug, and could prescribe the correct one right away. But unfortunately, there is no way to predict this. The same is true for hypertension. There are many different drugs belonging to various drug classes, but the doctor cannot predict with certainty which one will be effective. It is important that anyone contemplating taking an antidepressant medication for the first time realize that there is a good chance the first drug might not work, and they should be prepared to try a different drug if necessary. Their chances of eventually being significantly helped are very good.

Treatment Response and Cure

Initially, it was hoped that Prozac could make depressed people better than well, or at least completely cure them. I have seen patients with chronic, lifelong mild to moderate depressions feel better than they could ever remember. I have seen acute major depressive disorder patients smile and joke again as a result of their antidepressant treatment. But I have seen a fair number of partial improvements, patients who are once again able to sleep, eat, work, and participate in family life, but who still take little or no pleasure in life. They drag themselves through the day and collapse in bed at night. The depression is lessened, controlled, but not gone. I believe this is the reason why new antidepressant drugs continue to find a market among those whom the older drugs have not fully cured. I also am convinced this is why depressed people should never be treated by drugs alone, because too often these agents do not cure the patient. The psychiatrist must carefully evaluate the sufferer's overall functioning rather than settle for partial improvement with continued impairment, which can be addressed through psychotherapy.

CHAPTER 3

The Selective Serotonin Reuptake Inhibitors (SSRIs): Prozac, Zoloft, Paxil, and Luvox

Serotonin

Serotonin is one of the chemicals in the brain that transmits messages from one brain cell to another. It would be nice if the serotonin story were as simple as this: too little causes depression; too much, mania. But in fact, brain activities are controlled by the coming together of many different chemicals (also known as neurotransmitters), which serve as messengers from one cell to the next. Brain cells are excited not only by serotonin but also by norepinephrine, histamine, GABA, and acetylcholine, to name just a few. The interactions of the fifty-odd neurotransmitters with serotonin, therefore, involve serotonin in many brain activities that are disturbed in psychiatric symptoms and disorders, such as depression, anxiety, irritability, confused thinking, abnormal appetite, and disturbance of the sleep cycle. Furthermore, the neurotransmitters affect one another, and that may be why serotonin and nonserotonin antidepressants work equally well—when you give a drug affecting one neurotransmitter, you automatically affect the other neurotransmitters.

The term SSRI refers to selective serotonin reuptake inhibitor, a class of antidepressant drugs that are safer than, yet equally effective as, the older tricyclics. The SSRIs have mainly been researched in patients suffering from pure major depression and, to a lesser extent, in those suffering from obsessive-compulsive disorder and bulimia. Nearly every day, however, there are clinical reports of their effectiveness in the treatment of yet another condition. This seems to support the notion that there is a serotonin imbalance which crosses disease categories and explains this wide-ranging response. Because the SSRIs are safe drugs, and because the conditions they treat are serious, clinical necessity has forced their use before firm evidence of their effectiveness could be established. Anecdotal reports keep pouring in: the first known case of this or that, of a seventy-five-year-old stroke victim who cried for no reason being successfully cured by Zoloft, of two violent patients with different psychiatric conditions becoming much less aggressive after Zoloft. Later, I will list all the conditions to which the SSRIs have been applied with reported success, but with as yet insufficient scientific evidence. I do not wish to imply that these clinical efforts are in any way irresponsible. Physicians do not have complete and final evidence for much of what they do, some of which is much more serious than the mere prescribing of an SSRI. The example of the radical mastectomy comes to mind. When I was at Columbia University's College of Physicians and Surgeons from 1955 to 1959, the great Cushman Hagenson said emphatically that radical mastectomy was the only operation that could give a woman with breast cancer a chance at a full cure. Today, we know this is not the case. It seems he did not have all the evidence.

The SSRIs as a Class

More than half of all new antidepressant prescriptions written in the United States are for SSRIs. In the previous chapter, I called attention to their ease of use and their greater safety as being primarily responsible for their popularity. Because patients tolerate SSRIs better than the older antidepressants, more are able to complete an adequate dosage trial for a sufficient period of time to gain the full benefit of medication. A 1995 study noted that 60 percent of the severely depressed are treated by general practitioners who spend little time with these patients. They will give them a month's supply of SSRI at a time, instruct them to take one a day, and not worry too much about lethal overdose or about complicated side effects leading to noncompliance. Patients take these SSRIs daily and get better. The general doctor need not pay too much attention to them. Of course, there is some danger in inadequate medical supervision. The patient could have an unsuspected bipolar illness and be tipped over into mania by the SSRI. Furthermore, a study by A. C. Pande and M. E. Sayler (1993) of 3,183 outpatients in nineteen controlled studies of Prozac compared with a placebo or an older antidepressant found a remission rate in the severely depressed of only 27 to 29 percent on Prozac, 26 percent on a tricyclic antidepressant, and 18 percent on a placebo. These results are far from spectacular and demonstrate the need for the physician to carefully follow severely depressed patients and not merely send them off with a Prozac prescription in the naive belief that they will all get better. Once again, I must remind you of the difference between response (about 70 percent) and cure (found in this study to be only 27 to 29 percent). The improvement rate in the mild to moderately depressed as well as the cure rate, a Hamilton Depression score of 7 or less (see the previous chapter regarding Hamilton scores), is much better than in the severely depressed. But it is still far from perfect. People who are depressed, no matter how severely, need to be monitored closely for dose adjustment when necessary, and the doctor should check their medical status and psychiatric improvement and offer words of explanation, encouragement, and psychotherapy along with the drug. It would be nice if the scourge of depression could be completely resolved by a simple pill, new or old, SSRI or not, but this is far from always the case.

Nonetheless, the problems with the serotonin theory and the shortcomings of the SSRIs aside, these drugs have been very effective in treating the typical outpatient depressive. Safe and well-tolerated, they are usually effective taken once a day, often only a single pill. It is worth considering them together as a class before looking at their individual differences because they have much more in common than they have differences. Also, if after a trial of a month or two, there is little or no therapeutic response, it usually makes little sense to switch to another member of this same class for a second drug trial. Only when the first SSRI is effective but produces unacceptable side effects is use of another SSRI warranted. For example, if a patient becomes much less depressed on Prozac, but feels too tense, excited, and hyper, then a switch to Paxil, a more calming SSRI, makes sense.

The issue of classification of the twenty marketed antidepressants presents something of a problem. Some of the medicines are classified on the basis of their chemical structure (e.g., the tricyclics), some on the basis of their action on neurotransmitters (e.g., SSRIs), and some are not classified at all but listed simply as "other" (e.g., Wellbutrin). But in spite of this difficulty, it makes sense to use an antidepressant of a different class if the first one fails.

The SSRIs alter serotonin balance, but exactly what happens is not fully known. At first it was thought that by blocking reuptake they raised the level of available serotonin, but now it is known that the receptors are altered by becoming less sensitive. In any event, it is believed that serotonin is involved in the control of aggression, in sexual behavior, and in the maintenance of mood. The SSRIs, because of their effect on serotonin, have been used not only in depression but also in the following conditions:

Obsessive-compulsive disorder
Panic disorder
Bulimia and anorexia nervosa
Schizophrenia
Alcoholism
Borderline personality disorder
Autistic disorder
Impulsive aggressive behavior
Postpartum depression
Premenstrual syndrome
Social phobia
Pedophilia
Migraine headaches
Intermittent explosive disorder
Anxiety disorder

According to the evidence, their effectiveness ranges from excellent in depression, reasonably good in obsessive-compulsive disorder, and anecdotal in many of the other conditions. I am sure this list of SSRI uses is incomplete. Every day something new is added.

The SSRI Cure

Karen Jones, a forty-year-old married mother of one, had been unhappy in her marriage to John, her cold and uncaring husband, for almost all of the seven years they had been together. Not only did he not help with their four-year-old daughter, he seemed to avoid both of them, coming home from work as late as possible and going off to his study to hide and read. Karen felt lonely, angry, and unappreciated. She never smiled at John, refused sex except on the rarest occasions, and complained bitterly to him about his coldness and lack of cooperation in their family life.

Karen slept poorly, and appeared tired and grim. She stopped planning their social life and no longer read novels, previously her favorite activity. Karen had been seeing a therapist for two years. Much of the time they discussed her unhappy marriage, but she seemed unable to improve it. John refused to come to see the therapist with her, and Karen realized she could not fix her marriage alone. Besides, how could a withdrawn, cold engineer be transformed into a loving husband and father? Karen continued to worsen. She remained longer and longer in bed, returning to it as soon as she dropped her daughter off at preschool. She slept badly at night, started to lose weight, and stopped speaking to her friends and family. Her therapist, having become alarmed, suggested a psychopharmacology consult. A diagnosis of major depressive disorder was made, and she was given a prescription for Prozac. She asked the doctor why an SSRI and why the particular one she was suggesting. Her doctor said that all twenty antidepressants, old and new, had the same power to help her, that the newer ones had fewer side effects, and that of the eight newer ones, she had the most experience with the SSRIs. She decided to prescribe 10 mg of Prozac each morning, half the typical 20-mg starting dose, because some people could not tolerate the larger amount right away. The doctor said she had chosen Prozac over Paxil, Zoloft, or Luvox because it had been available since 1988, and its faults and dangers were more likely to be known than those of the other, newer members of the SSRI class.

She added that the other SSRIs had some advantages. They were less activating, so that people felt less "wired" and nervous on them, but diarrhea was slightly more frequent with Zoloft, while dry mouth and drowsiness were more likely with Paxil. All the SSRIs cause insomnia, which can often be overcome by taking the drug in the morning or by lowering the dose. Nausea is also a problem with the SSRIs, which can be lessened by taking the medicine with meals and tends to dis-

appear after several weeks. Common to all SSRIs and estimated to afflict between 30 and 40 percent (some experts say
up to 80 percent) of users is sexual dysfunction in both men
and women. The doctor went on to say that although the
eight new antidepressants were all as effective as the twelve
older ones and caused fewer side effects, none of them were
perfect.

One week later, Karen returned for a follow-up visit, saying
she was sleeping a little better, and she appeared less grim
and tired. Otherwise, nothing had changed. She continued to
spend too much time in bed. The psychopharmacologist
asked about side effects and, discovering none, raised the
Prozac dose to 20 mg. Two weeks later, on her return visit,
Karen said she felt a little nervous and had a little diarrhea,
but that neither was excessive. What had changed was that she
was no longer spending the day in bed. In fact, she had been
to lunch with several of her friends and had had a good time.
She did not feel up to books yet, but had read several magazines and had gone to a lecture she enjoyed. On each of her
biweekly visits over the next several months, she reported slow
but steady improvement, until, after the fourth month of
treatment, she told the psychopharmacologist something the
doctor considered quite remarkable. Karen had had a talk
with her husband in which she discovered he had been quite
angry at her for what he perceived as her laziness and lack of
attention to him and the child. His perception had been that
he did all the work outside the home and then came back to
do everything inside it as well. He was less angry now that
Karen had gotten out of bed and begun to straighten up their
home and their marriage. He enjoyed sex with her for the
first time in years, in spite of his understanding that Prozac
hampered her responsiveness. Most of all, John said, he felt
once again, for the first time in years, that Karen loved rather
than hated him, and he once again enjoyed being with her.
Indeed, John began coming home earlier from work and
enjoyed the company of his wife and daughter.

Karen reported that she understood the effect of her

depression on her husband, how her lack of energy and anger had made him withdraw warily from her. She was fully aware that what she gave in her marriage was what she got; that if she was good to John, he would be kind to her. She also marveled at how this simple recognition had eluded her in her years of therapy. In fact, the sympathy of her therapist regarding how hard it was for her to be married to this cold, withdrawn man implied that he had caused her depression, rather than merely responding to and suffering because of it.

How Effective Are the SSRIs?

Every antidepressant treatment, including the SSRIs, older antidepressants, and even electroshock, affects serotonin neurotransmission. All the SSRIs are equal in efficacy to all the older and newer antidepressant drugs, but they have fewer side effects. The reason for this lies in the word *selective* in selective serotonin reuptake inhibitors. While the ability to tolerate SSRIs better than older antidepressants is of enormous importance, the hope that they would cure more patients has not been realized. In general, there is no one group of depressives or patients who benefit more from an SSRI than from other antidepressant drugs. Furthermore, the SSRIs do not cure patients more rapidly than other antidepressants. With all the antidepressants, there is a five-day to three-week or longer wait before improvement occurs.

The SSRIs have proven to be as effective as older antidepressants in the treatment of severe depression. Unfortunately, as I mentioned earlier, while the response rate in severe depression is not too bad, the cure rate is low and slow for the SSRIs. These are wonderful drugs, but they are not miracle drugs. Patients with severe depression must tolerate weeks and months of waiting before they truly feel better.

Of All the Antidepressants, Old and New, Should the SSRIs Be Used First?

Judging by the number of prescriptions written, most physicians and psychiatrists prescribe SSRIs first. The SSRIs are as effective as any of the others and have the fewest side effects. Most people tolerate them well and are able to complete a full course of treatment. They only have to be taken once a day, which is easy to remember. Most of the time, one pill is all that is needed, which makes frequent trips to the doctor for dose adjustment unnecessary. Because they have been prescribed so widely, many of their few bad secrets have been revealed. Brand-new drugs pose unknown risks.

The SSRIs are the antidepressants I use first, and often second, too, if the first one fails or cannot be tolerated. It is only then that I will turn to a newer or older agent. Most physicians seem to do the same.

Depression Combined with Anxiety

Many depressed patients also suffer from anxiety. Anxiety affects both mind and body, causing gloomy and fearful thoughts, along with rapid pulse, sweaty palms, and abdominal symptoms. Whether one causes the other or both are produced by something else is unknown. What is known is that a patient with a major depressive disorder is more than ten times as likely to develop an anxiety disorder either simultaneously or in the future. Perhaps this is further evidence for the serotonin or neurotransmitter imbalance I spoke of earlier, since serotonin may play a role in both anxiety and depression. Various theories notwithstanding, many physicians were concerned about prescribing an SSRI to depressed patients who were also anxious or prone to anxiety since one prominent side effect of these new medications is an increase in anxiety, especially early in treatment. These physicians reasoned that a sedating antidepressant such as Elavil or Serzone would be a better choice. This clinical "logic" has proven incorrect. Ironically, anxiety can be a side effect of the SSRIs, yet they are better than the older sedating antidepressants in the treatment of anxiety accompanied by depression. In addition, the SSRIs act faster, and are also effective in panic disorders.

Suicidal Preoccupation

Contrary to an early false report, the SSRIs do *not* cause or worsen suicidal thoughts or behavior. Unfortunately, as with all other antidepressants, SSRIs are not effective in 30 percent of patients, and the failure figure is higher in severe depressives. Suicidal thoughts and attempts occur during SSFL therapy at the same rate as they do during tricyclic antidepressant treatment, but overdose deaths are much lower from the new drugs than the old ones. When compared to a placebo, SSRLs lessen suicidal thoughts and actions. Furthermore, no deaths have occurred from the overdose of an SSRI alone, although there have been some when the drug was taken along with other medications and alcohol. When taken in overdose, Prozac causes nausea, vomiting, and restlessness, and Zoloft and Paxil overdoses cause drowsiness and a slowed pulse rate.

Switches into Mania

Occasionally, a depressed person turns into a manic one. On the rare occasions when this happens, the consequences can be very serious and the patient may require hospitalization. When someone is a known bipolar (manic-depressive), this danger can be guarded against with medication. Sometimes, however, this occurs unexpectedly. The question of whether such events are caused by the antidepressant medication or whether the person was simply due to have a manic episode is difficult to settle in an individual instance. A few studies and several experts have found that the SSRIs are associated with manic switches in 1 percent of cases whereas the tricyclics are responsible in 2 percent. They recommend shorter-duration SSRIs like Paxil so that if the manic episode is induced, use of the drug can be stopped without lingering effects. Over the years, I have found the manic switch to be very rare in depressed outpatients without a history of mania or hypomania and who have no manic-depressive relatives. On the rare occasion when it does happen, it is best spotted by a friend, relative, or doctor since the patient may suffer a loss of judgment and be unaware of what is happening.

SSRIs are effective in known bipolar depressed people who are taking lithium, Tegretol, or Depakote. They may be used safely and in the normal dosage.

Dysthymic Disorder

Dys means "bad" and *thymia* means "mind" or "soul" in Latin. Dysthymic disorder lies on the border between the normal and the pathologic, and that border is engulfed in fog. The official psychiatric diagnostic manual has attempted to clear that fog three times in the last fourteen years (1980, 1987, 1994) without great success. The psychiatric microscope remains uncleaned and without power to tell us what is the normal level of suffering associated with the human condition and what is pathologic. It currently defines dysthymic disorder as a "chronically depressed mood" present for most of two years or longer, and accompanied by changes in appetite, sleep, and energy along with low self-esteem, poor concentration, difficulty making decisions, and feelings of hopelessness. An individual need have only two of the ten items listed in addition to a chronic bad mood, so many different combinations of symptoms are possible. For example, if someone feels sad and is overweight and without much energy, that person is dysthymic. Another individual may feel down, have difficulty concentrating at his job, and have low

self-esteem. He, too, is dysthymic. Someone else may have
trouble sleeping and making decisions and feel down in the
dumps. She, too, is dysthymic. Another individual may sleep
too much, eat too little, and feel depressed. The question of
who has the illness dysthymic disorder, requiring a drug, and
who is not sick but needs to change his life in order to feel
better can be a difficult one for doctor and patient.

The concept of dysthymia and the efforts to objectively
depict it arise out of a desire to make psychiatry scientifically
valid and objectively capable of studying its illnesses and treatments. The observable symptom list of dysthymia replaces the
concept of neurosis with its hidden, unconscious desires and
conflicts, largely inferred by psychoanalytic believers and difficult to see for nonbelievers. Dysthymic patients are the "neu-
rotics" of twenty years ago, and the people who now take care
of them would like to be able to agree with one another
regarding their diagnosis and treatment.

The problem for psychiatry is shared by all of medicine.
There are the very sick, the well, and all those in the ill-
defined middle. The cancer doctor has the same difficulty: he
or she tries to grade cancer 1, 2, 3, 3b, 4, 4b, or 5, in order to
tell what will happen to the patient or how long she will live.
Grade 1 may be very slow-growing and grade 5 overwhelmingly fast, but the numbers in the middle may not mean
much. Some dysthymics are quite dysfunctional, drag themselves to work if they are even able to do that, but otherwise
lie in bed or sit on a couch. They have few social contacts, no
hobbies or interests, and exist from day to day without goals
or pleasure. The healthy dysthymics are lawyers or surgeons
who work all the time, do not smile much, are over- or under-
weight, and may have trouble making decisions or falling
asleep. Are they sick or merely grim? The sick dysthymics
often have episodes of major depression. Do they have two
diseases (so-called double depression) or is it a varying
expression of the same illness? The healthy dysthymics continue on in their plodding, workaholic ways. The analogy with
cancer grading applies—those with mild forms will probably

die of something unrelated. The questions as to which cancerous prostates to remove and which to leave untreated until old age or some other condition leads to death continue to be debated. Almost all agree that something ought to be done about the severe cases of cancer, and similarly of dysthymia. A 1995 article published in the *American Journal of Psychiatry* adds to the complexity of dysthymia. The authors found that lifelong dysthymics are much more inclined than those people with episodic major depression to have borderline, histrionic, self-defeating, dependent, or avoidant personalities. The researchers refused to take a position on whether the personality disorder caused or was a result of the dysthymia, or whether both were due to some unknown reason. But the study once again shows the link between illness and personality and the difficulty of separating one from the other.

SSRIs help dysthymics, but almost all the evidence is anecdotal. These are the people who have been depressed since childhood, who Peter Kramer, author of *Listening to Prozac*, reported felt "better than well" on Prozac. Most psychopharmacologists and psychiatrists (including myself) think not that the drug gave them an artificial high, but that it removed their depressive features, allowing their self-esteem to rise, along with their energy and mood, so that they could function in a healthy way for the first time. Many of these people had been in psychotherapy for years with varying degrees of benefit, but Prozac made a profound difference. I have seen this phenomenon occur in my practice, sometimes after having worked with the person in psychotherapy without drugs for several years. An SSRI lifted the person's confidence, helped him organize his thoughts, gave him the courage to speak before a group, helped him become more active in the community, and brightened his outlook on life. Some who never expected anything good to ever happen began to plan optimistically.

The writings on dysthymia regarding drug treatment come mostly from those who have observed the sick end of the dysthymic spectrum, those who describe the frequency of major depressive episodes in this group. My own experience with outpatient, functioning dysthymics has made diagnosis much more difficult than it is for those who deal with the sickest end of the condition. On the healthier side, they are limited in their occupational, social, and family functioning, yet it is not so easy to say whether they are experiencing normal human suffering or dysthymic disorder. I tell such people about the SSRIs and explain that my capacity to guide them is limited. It is up to them to decide whether their suffering has gone beyond the edge of normal. Most decide to do without the drug. Of those who try, a large majority feel much better, and the quality of their lives improves. Occasionally, I run into a drug-type who will ingest anything for a new experience, or to achieve a high, but most of my patients are not that way. They are sincerely trying to help themselves and their friends and families. I trust these people to make their own diagnosis with the help of my limited knowledge.

I think it will be a long time before science will be able to define accurately and cure dysthymia. The condition is chronic, hard to diagnose, and frequently difficult to treat. The diagnostic criteria keep changing because of advancing knowledge, and the changes present a problem for the study of a chronic illness. Studies begun years ago are no longer valid for current purposes of diagnosis. This is particularly problematic for a vague condition like dysthymia, but even what I called schizophrenia during my residency in the early 1960s is no longer considered schizophrenia. Does this mean the drug studies of that era no longer apply?

I leave you with my conviction, shared by many of my colleagues, that if you suffer from dysthymia and it interferes with your work and your relationships with your children, friends, family, and lovers, and if therapy has helped to some extent, but not enough, try an SSRI. It could make a huge difference for you.

If Side Effects Force You to Stop One SSRI, Will You Be Able to Tolerate Another?

Drs. Walter Brown and Wilma Harrison questioned 113 patients with major depression (*Journal of Clinical Psychiatry*, January 1995) who had discontinued Prozac because of side effects. The side effects most commonly causing patients to stop taking the drug were insomnia, agitation, anxiety, headache, sleepiness, nervousness, fatigue, decreased libido, impaired concentration, and nausea. A month after stopping Prozac, they were started on Zoloft. Seventy-nine percent of the patients completed Zoloft treatment, and only 10 percent discontinued because of side effects. The patients completed several months of Zoloft treatment in spite of gastrointestinal symptoms, insomnia, sexual dysfunction, somnolence, and agitation. One shortcoming of this study is that it was not double-blind—that is, it did not give half of the patients Prozac again and the other half Zoloft without telling them which one they were getting. In spite of this, it seems to make the point that if one cannot tolerate Prozac, another SSRI may do. My personal clinical experience corroborates this fact. People who cannot tolerate one SSRI frequently respond well to another.

SSRI Use During Psychoanalysis

During my Harvard psychiatric residency more than thirty years ago, one of my professors, Dr. Elvin Semrad, a legendary psychoanalytic teacher in Boston, required us to stop medicating our patients before he interviewed them so that their heads would not be disconnected from their bodies and he could discover what really bothered them—the feelings they found it so difficult or impossible to tolerate. The psychoanalyst of that era did not medicate the psychoanalytic neurotic and was extremely reluctant to give drugs even to the dangerous, hospitalized, paranoid schizophrenic. Drugs were slipped to the latter in a "don't ask, don't tell" manner. In fact, 60 percent of the hospitalized patients were on tranquilizers or antidepressants, but no one made a great point of this embarrassing statistic to Dr. Semrad. I give you this bit of history so you can share my surprise when I read an article by Drs. Stephen Donovan and Steven Roose in the May 1995 issue of the *Journal of Clinical Psychiatry*. Donovan and Roose surveyed forty-five training analysts at the Columbia University Center for Psychoanalytic Training and Research and discovered that 18 percent of 277 patients in analysis were on a psychiatric drug, that most of them were depressed and on an SSRI, and that both the patient's mood and the analytic process improved. They noted that this contradicts "the belief that medication undermines the psychoanalytic situation." If Dr. Semrad is watching from heaven, he just learned something. But there are still psychotherapists of the old school who resist the idea of their clients and patients taking SSRIs or other psychoactive drugs. If you are currently seeing a physician like this, I suggest you tactfully urge a psychopharmacological consult. If the SSRI-resister is your family doctor and he or she lectures you about willpower, but willpower repeatedly fails you so that you cannot get yourself to do the thing you know you need to do—such as talk to your children, perform with more energy at work, be nice to your spouse, or call your friends—then I suggest you tell your family practitioner you want to see a psychiatrist for evaluation and possible SSRI treatment, and that willpower may work for him or her, but you are sick and need treatment.

Is It Safe to Switch from Prozac to Paxil Without Waiting Two Weeks in Between?

Margaret Kreider, Ph.D., of SmithKline Beecham Pharmaceuticals, et al. studied the switch from Prozac to Paxil in two groups of over 100 patients each, one of which was switched from Prozac to Paxil immediately, and the other of which had two weeks of a placebo in between. They found that the switch was equally well tolerated by both groups (*Journal of Clinical Psychiatry*, April 1995). Since Prozac remains in the blood for several weeks after its use is discontinued, many people are concerned about switching from Prozac to Paxil without waiting at least two weeks. As I have noted before, over 40 percent of depressed patients do not get better on the first drug given, either because of an inability to tolerate the side effects or because the drug fails to work. Therefore, questions of when and how to switch to another antidepressant are not academic but of practical, clinical importance. The changeovers must be considered carefully since some are dangerous and require a washout period in which no drug is given. The switch from Prozac to Paxil is not one of these.

Discontinuing Use of SSRIs

Since Prozac is a long-acting drug that remains in the blood for weeks, the changeover from it to Paxil is tolerated, even though it is sudden. Nonetheless, discontinuing use of SSRIs is best done gradually in order to spare patients unnecessary upset. I have observed what Dr. James Ellison calls a "withdrawal buzz," a painful "shock" in the head (also described as a "jolt" or "rush") in people who suddenly stop taking an SSRI. Why this occurs is unknown, but what is known is that it is not dangerous to the brain, and patients do not faint because of it. It is unpleasant, though, and can be avoided by very gradually tapering off use of the drug. Sometimes, as in the event of a severe allergic reaction to the drug, there is no choice, and use of the SSRI must be stopped suddenly. Any ill effects can be handled by an unrelated medication, but often there is no need.

Social Phobia and the SSRIs

The *Diagnostic and Statistical Manual* (4th ed., 1994) of the American Psychiatric Association defines social phobia as a "marked and persistent fear of one or more social or performance situations in which the person is exposed to unfamiliar people or to possible scrutiny by others." The person is in fear of humiliating or embarrassing himself, and either avoids such situations or endures them with anxiety. The avoidance and intense anxiety interferes with the person's work, school, and/or social life. The condition can either be generalized, as in extreme shyness and avoidance, or be confined to one area, such as public speaking.

Considering that it is estimated that 20 million Americans will become social phobics sometime in their lifetime, and that this would make it the third most common psychiatric condition after major depressive episodes and alcohol dependence, remarkably little is known about it. Twice as many women as men have it, often since early adolescence. In fact, 80 percent of cases occur before age twenty-five, and because it is chronic, it severely interferes with the person's life, since they avoid speaking in front of groups or to strangers, meeting new people, or eating in public. As a result, according to Dr. Lewis Judd, two thirds of social phobics are unmarried, half never completed high school, and 20 percent are unable to work. Unlike agoraphobics, who avoid places for fear of having a panic attack, social phobics avoid situations where they may be evaluated, ridiculed, or humiliated. It is believed, based on studies, that genetic factors play an important role.

An article by Dr. Randall Marshall in the *Journal of Clinical Psychiatry* (June 1994) quotes two figures for the odds of suffering social phobia within one's lifetime: 2.4 percent and 13.3 percent. One figure is more than five times the other. No wonder efforts to find biological markers for the condition have been unsuccessful. Clearly, it is poorly defined. Jerome

Kagan, who has studied shyness, describes a severe type of social phobia resulting in rapid pulse and overwhelming anxiety when a child is separated from its mother and confronted with new situations. But Dr. Kagan also describes a more moderate type of social phobia, one that can be overcome at a cocktail party filled with strangers by the simple downing of a first drink.

In spite of the lack of solid, scientific, objective criteria acceptable to all authorities as the cause and basis for cure of social phobia, I have seen this condition repeatedly during my psychiatric career, and watched it destroy many people's lives. The woman who is lonely and wants to meet men, but cannot bring herself to meet people who may judge and/or ridicule her, continues to sit at home alone. The graduate student who is terrified every time he goes to class that the professor might call on him. The consultant who cannot sleep the night before he makes a presentation before a client and becomes tongue-tied and does badly. The member of the symphony orchestra who shakes so badly she cannot play. The student who cannot give his oral report or who freezes during an examination. Social phobia is a real condition, a terrible condition, and one that ruins lives, but it is also a mild condition, something we all feel to some extent in the presence of strangers, in front of audiences, when we are going to be judged. At worst, it is a terrible affliction that can ruin lives. At best, it can be a source of mild social discomfort. If you think you have social phobia and have been losing out on your life, you should consult a psychotherapist and consider taking one of the following drugs:

B-adrenergic blockers
   propranolol (Inderal)
   atenolol (Tenormin)
   nadolol (Corgard)
Monoamine oxidase inhibitors
   phenelzine (Nardil)
   tranylcypromine (Parnate)

Benzodiazepines
  clonazepam (Klonopin)
  alprazolam (Xanax)
SSRIs—Prozac, Zoloft, Paxil, Luvox
Buspirone (Buspar)

Inderal is the well-known stage-fright drug that stops the motor manifestations of anxiety such as hand-shaking, sweating, and racing pulse. It is taken by musicians and actors. It is sometimes handed out without a prescription by theater directors, which is not a good idea, since it should not be taken by asthmatics and can dangerously lower the blood pressure. Clearly, a doctor's supervision is called for. Inderal should be taken twenty to thirty minutes before a performance, such as public speaking, playing a stringed instrument, or exercising a skill in public that requires a steady hand. Tenormin and Corgard, which are prescribed less often, work similarly to Inderal. In generalized social phobia, which occurs in all social situations, as opposed to only a few circumstances, B-blockers are of no use.

The MAOIs (monoamine oxidase inhibitors) Nardil and Parnate are effective in the treatment of generalized social phobias, decreasing a person's excessive sensitivity to being viewed and judged. The problem with the MAOIs is their side effects and the dietary restrictions necessitated by their use. It is hoped that the much less problematic SSRIs (to be described next) will be equally effective in treating generalized social phobics, but controlled studies remain to be done. In the office and anecdotally, the SSRIs seem fine. An experimental MAOI, Moclobemide, which is easier and safer to use than Nardil and Parnate, may be released by the Food and Drug Administration soon, and prove useful in the treatment of social phobics.

Buspirone, an antianxiety agent with serotonin effects, may also be of some use, but there is considerable doubt about its efficacy in social phobia.

The antianxiety agents Xanax and Klonopin are of help in

treating generalized social phobia, as are behavior and cognitive therapies.

The SSRIs (Prozac, Zoloft, Paxil, and Luvox) have all been used to treat social phobia. They have been found effective in the studies done, but these have been open, as opposed to double-blind placebo-controlled, which means they are flawed because both the researcher and the patient knew that an SSRI was being given, and their expectations may have colored the results.

Once again, the borders of social phobia present a research and therapeutic problem. Not only is there the border between normal stranger anxiety and excessive fear, but there is the border with other psychiatric conditions. Most social phobics also have either panic disorder, simple phobia, or obsessive-compulsive disorder. Furthermore, many are depressed because of their narrow lives, lack of confidence, and perhaps because whatever it is that makes them avoid new people and situations also makes them depressed. High sensitivity to rejection exists in both social phobics and depressives. MAOIs and SSRIs reduce this interpersonal hypersensitivity, allowing the individual to care less about what others may think and thus to go out into the world.

Obsessive-Compulsive Disorder (OCD)

Obsessive-compulsive disorder is characterized by obsessions and compulsions that are usually chronic. Obsessions refer to recurrent and unwanted thoughts that cause anxiety and discomfort because of their aggressive, sexual, or disgusting content. They include such things as fear of dirt and harm to the self or others. OCD patients are plagued by doubt about whether their hands are clean or the door is locked. Compulsions are behaviors such as hand-washing and checking the stove or door lock. OCD is not to be confused with compulsive personality. The OCD patient suffers from a compulsion that must be resisted, whereas the obsessive-

compulsive personality disorder patient is happy in his orderliness and stinginess. The former rarity and now commonness
(a lifetime rate of 2.5 percent) of OCD is attributed to these
patients' secretiveness about their symptoms. To determine if
you have OCD, ask yourself whether you have repetitive
thoughts that seem horrible or weird, or things you do over
and over again.

A 1984 National Epidemiologic Catchment Area (ECA)
survey found that OCD was fifty to one hundred times more
common than previously believed, affecting 1 to 2 percent of
the population worldwide, and making it the fourth most
common psychiatric disorder (after phobias, substance abuse,
and major depression). There are two problems with this
finding. One is that lay interviewers were used, and second,
even more importantly, no careful evaluation of how the
symptoms impaired the OCD sufferers was made. However,
other studies have addressed these shortcomings, and found
OCD to be as common as the ECA survey showed. Patients
with OCD are more likely to also have schizophrenia, depression, Tourette's syndrome (involuntary muscle tics and vocal
tics including obscene words), and other anxiety disorders.

The SSRIs have become the primary treatment for OCD,
along with the tricyclic clomipramine. Serotonin has been
studied in OCD and is found to have a role, as it does in
aggression, anxiety, learning, social dominance, impulsivity,
and suicide. Clomipramine has a potent serotonin effect, and
is more effective against OCD than is desipramine, which is a
norepinephrine-specific tricyclic. All the SSRIs have proved
effective in treating OCD and, combined with behavior
therapy, offer those suffering from this painful and debilitating condition real hope of spending less time obsessing,
checking, hoarding, and washing, and more time with family,
friends, and in meaningful work. This combination therapy
helps most people get a lot better, but does not cure them
completely. Because OCD is a chronic illness that waxes and
wanes, SSRI treatment must be long-term. Symptomatic
improvement may continue steadily for months.

Panic Disorder and the SSRIs

Panic disorder is a condition consisting of recurrent, spontaneous attacks of intense fear accompanied by some or all of the following: palpitations, sweating, shaking, shortness of breath, a choking feeling, chest pain, nausea, dizziness, numbness, chills, hot flashes, and feelings of unreality, of going crazy, or of dying. Panic attacks can be caused by a specific or social phobia or by post-traumatic stress disorder (a flashback), or they can be unexpected. In panic disorder, patients suddenly and unexpectedly feel faint, their hearts pound, they fear they will die, and they have difficulty breathing. They are often young adults who have recently experienced one of the following: the death of a loved one, a life-threatening illness or accident, separation from their family, thyroid disease, the birth of a child, or the taking of a mind-altering drug. Many panic disorder patients had school phobia as children.

Tricyclic antidepressants have been repeatedly demonstrated in carefully conducted controlled trials to stop panic attacks in patients who are not depressed. Imipramine, a tricyclic antidepressant highly effective in treating panic disorder, is also used in children with school phobia, making them able to leave their mothers and go to school. Imipramine does not stop the patient's fear of the next attack. This so-called anticipatory anxiety may require a benzodiazepine such as Valium, Ativan, or Klonopin. MAOIs and other tricyclic antidepressants also block panic attacks.

The SSRIs are also very effective in the treatment of panic. Like Imipramine, Prozac can also overstimulate panic patients if started at the usual 20-mg dose. To avoid this, the drug is started at 5 mg a day and raised 5 mg every week until 20 mg is reached, which is usually enough. The panic attacks are usually controlled within four to twelve weeks. It is not known exactly how long someone will have to stay on antidepressant drug therapy to prevent recurrence of panic attacks. Since it is a chronic disorder that improves and relapses, the therapy may have to go on a long time.

The benzodiazepines Xanax and Klonopin have also proved effective in the treatment of panic. Studies are under way comparing them with the antidepressants. They have fewer initial side effects than antidepressants, act faster, and are also effective against fear of the next attack, but because they pose some danger of dependence and withdrawal, their use is reserved until antidepressants fail. Most psychopharmacologists believe that the problem of addiction to benzodiazepines (Valium, Xanax, Ativan, etc.) has been exaggerated, and applies to addicts rather than the general population, which is able to stop taking them when they are no longer needed without serious consequences.

Side Effects of the SSRIs

Nausea without vomiting, loose stools and diarrhea, nervousness and anxiety, loss of appetite, insomnia, headache, and sexual dysfunction are all potential side effects of the SSRIs. As treatment continues, many of the side effects go away, especially nausea and headache. Some of the symptoms, such as anxiety, headache, loss of sex drive, and abdominal distress, are due to the depression itself, and not to the drug. In general, the higher the dose of the drug, the more side effects. It therefore makes sense to start at as low a dosage as possible and move up gradually. Antidepressants work slowly, taking days to weeks, and the tendency to increase the dosage instead of waiting for the therapeutic effect causes more side effects than are necessary. When side effects do occur, the dose can be reduced or divided or taken at a different time of day, another antidepressant can be tried, or the side effects can be treated.

Nausea

This can be a problem with any of the SSRIs, but if the drug is taken with food or the dose decreased, it is tolerable. After a few weeks, nausea disappears. About 25 percent of people on SSRIs become nauseous, but only 5 percent have to discontinue the drug because of it. If nausea or vomiting becomes excessive, the gastric agent cisapride is effective in stopping it, but it must be used cautiously because of danger to the heart, when combined with Serzone and several non-antidepressants.

Insomnia

All the SSRIs cause insomnia in about 20 percent of those who take them. This can be minimized by taking the drug in the morning and, if this fails, lessening the dose until the symptom disappears, in which case the dose can be raised again. Sometimes the insomnia is due not to the SSRI but to worsening depression, drug-caused muscle restlessness, or mania. If the insomnia continues, an additional sedating antidepressant can be prescribed, such as trazodone (Desyrel, etc.), or a benzodiazepine, such as triazolam (Halcion), at bedtime.

Nervousness and Anxiety

Especially at the beginning of treatment, about 20 percent of people feel "wired," jittery, restless, irritable, and shaky. It may be due to the SSRI, or to worsening depression, incipient mania, or drug-induced motor restlessness. If it is due to the SSRI, dose reduction and waiting to get used to the drug often works. Then the dose can be raised gradually. If the "wired" feeling continues, the drug can be changed to another antidepressant, or an antianxiety drug like Valium or Ativan be added.

Headache

Headache is a very common symptom of major depression. SSRIs may induce or exacerbate tension and migraine headaches. In fact, SSRIs cause more headaches than do the older tricyclic antidepressants. As with other side effects, alternative causes of headache must be considered and ruled out. The dosage can be reduced while the patient gets used to the drug; changes in diet, exercise, and stress reduction can be advised, aspirin taken as needed, or small doses of Elavil added.

Weight Gain

The SSRIs are certainly better than the older antidepressants regarding weight gain. Most people are able to undergo a full course of treatment without gaining a pound. Occasionally, a person on an SSRI will gain a lot of weight. This may be due to untreated depression, since some depressives overeat, and many are underactive. Sometimes weight gain is due to thyroid dysfunction.

I advise people on SSRIs to watch the scale regularly, to exercise, and to seek nutritional counseling should their weight increase. Occasionally, the addition of the stimulants Dexedrine or Ritalin to the SSRI will increase the antidepressant effect and decrease weight. The overwhelming majority of the people I have treated do not end up abusing the Dexedrine or Ritalin when it is used for this purpose, but many drugstores, because of governmental harassment and fear of break-ins, no longer stock Dexedrine.

Hypomania and Mania

Every antidepressant can be associated with mania, but whether the drug actually causes it or otherwise unearths it in individuals who would become manic anyway is an ongoing debate among experts. If you are taking an SSRI and you suddenly feel extraordinarily happy, your thoughts begin to race, you sleep only a couple of hours a night, you have boundless energy, you start to spend money you do not have, and you begin to engage in business activities and romantic liaisons that horrify your friends and family, then use of the antidepressant must be stopped immediately and the doctor called right away. If you have only a mild version and feel just a little speeded up and unable to sleep, a dosage reduction may be all you need.

If you know you are bipolar (manic-depressive) or have relatives who are, be sure to tell your doctor before starting an SSRI. But if you are an outpatient dysthymic or other depressive type who needs an SSRI, you probably have little reason to worry that it will suddenly make you manic.

Drowsiness

About 20 percent of people on SSRIs feel drugged or drowsy, and about 5 percent discontinue use of the drug because of it. Although less frequent than with the older tricyclics, it can still be a problem. Sometimes drowsiness is due to the SSRI-induced insomnia, but often not. If drowsiness occurs, it is best to take the drug in the evening, and if this fails, to lower the dose. Also, try an extra cup of coffee in the morning.

Sexual Dysfunction

Disturbances in sexual functioning have emerged as the principal problem with the SSRIs and have caused many people to stop taking them, often at the risk of becoming depressed again. Initially reported in the *Physicians' Desk Reference (PDR)* as a low occurrence rate, it is now estimated at 30 to 50 percent or higher. The reason it was initially missed is that there is no requirement that drug-induced sexual difficulties be a topic of questioning in prerelease drug trials. If not asked, people, particularly women, are not likely to mention them, especially when they are being treated for major depression.

The sexual difficulties caused by the SSRIs include: decrease or absence of sexual desire; delayed, painful, or absence of orgasm; and erectile dysfunction.

While it is necessary to remember that sexual problems are widespread in the general population, and that diminished desire is certainly common in the depressed (and is, in fact, one factor in its diagnosis), there is no question that SSRI-induced sexual difficulties are a major problem, causing people not to want to take the drug, and to stop taking it when they should not.

Take the case of Barbara. She loved sex with her husband throughout the eighteen years of their marriage. While their relationship had otherwise been stormy as they struggled on limited funds to bring up their children, their bedroom was their salvation. Unfortunately, there was major depression in Barbara's family, and she, too, had had numerous episodes of it, never requiring hospitalization, but nonetheless quite debilitating. She would be confined to her bed for days at a time, get headaches, backaches, and stomach problems, and lose days at work. Fortunately, antidepressants had helped her over the years, but the tricyclics had made her gain weight, which she struggled in vain to lose. Barbara welcomed the SSRIs because of their reputation of not causing users to put on poundage. But they ruined her desire and her capacity for orgasm. As soon as she recovered from her latest episode of depression, she stopped taking them, even though she realized she had a good chance of getting depressed again. It was not long before this happened.

A growing list of ways to cope with the SSRI sexual side effect is largely anecdotal and may be effective. The simplest is dose reduction and waiting for the problem to go away, but this is far from always what happens. People taking Zoloft or Paxil (this does not work with long-acting Prozac) can skip the drug a day or two before anticipated sexual activity. The second is switching to Wellbutrin or Serzone, with continued antidepressant effect and normalization of sexual function. If these latter two antidepressants were as good as the SSRIs in every other way and had fewer or no sexual side effects, then the issue could easily be resolved by people taking them in the first place and skipping the SSRIs; but these drugs have other detriments (discussed in Chapter 4) so the SSRIs remain the first choice among most psychiatrists. But once the SSRI sexual side effect gets out of hand, this may be a sensible alternative. Short of stopping use of the SSRIs because of sexual side effects, a variety of drugs have been tried to reverse the problem. The reports of their success are anecdotal and not well studied. They include:

Bethanechol (Urecholine, etc.)

Taken thirty minutes to two hours before sexual activity, bethanechol has been shown to be effective in overcoming sexual dysfunction. It is not to be taken by patients with asthma, ulcers, or cardiac disease, and can worsen diarrhea induced by the SSRIs, as well as causing a running nose, excessive tearing, and stomach cramps. A similar drug (neostigmine) can also be used.

Yohimbine (Yocon, Yohimex, etc.)

Taken two to four hours before intercourse, yohimbine seems to correct all sexual problems, including lack of desire, arousal, orgasm, and ejaculation, but the studies have been open rather than double-blind controlled, and require verification. The dosage seems somewhat difficult to adjust since too little does no good, and too much makes people feel shaky, wired, anxious, or tense. Nonetheless, it seems to work pretty well, and I have tried it in a few patients with success. Other yohimbine side effects include nausea, increased heart rate, blood pressure, and irritability, but they are usually not serious. While the *PDR* may be overly cautious in warning against its use in females or in psychiatric patients, my experience has been that it works well in both. The *PDR* further warns that the drug should not be used with antidepressants, which may be true for the tricyclics, but not for the SSRIs. The *PDR* warns against the use of yohimbine in pregnant women and anyone suffering from renal disease or gastric ulcers.

Cyproheptadine (Periactin, etc.)

Cyproheptadine is an antiserotonin antihistamine that has been used to reverse SSRI sexual dysfunction. I have resisted using it because it can reverse the antidepressant effect of the SSRIs. Drugs that raise the level of serotonin in the brain lower the sex drive.

Dopamine

The neurotransmitter dopamine has been shown to increase male sexual behavior in rats, and drugs that increase the level of dopamine have been observed to increase penile erection. It has been reported that Parkinson patients on levodopa, a drug converted to dopamine in the body and used to treat parkinsonism, have increased libido, spontaneous erections, and nocturnal emissions. Because of these reports, several dopamine-raising drugs have been tried to relieve SSRI-induced sexual dysfunction. They are:

Amantadine
Dextroamphetamine
Pemoline (Cylert)
Bromocriptine (Parlodel)

Central Serotonin Syndrome (CSS)

When an SSRI and an MAOI (Nardil, Parnate, etc.) are administered together or within two to five weeks of each another, central serotonin syndrome (CSS) can occur. Characterized by fever, sweating, rapid pulse, high blood pressure, rigidity, confusion, and disturbed consciousness, it can result in coma or death. Unless mixed with another serotonin-elevating drug, the SSRIs do not cause CSS, and are safe.

Sweating and Dry Mouth

Sweating and dry mouth are not common problems with the SSRIs, but they do occur. Dry mouth can be combated with sugar-free gum and candies and drops of artificial saliva. Dental caries should be guarded against by careful mouth hygiene.

Some increase in sweating, especially in the upper body, may occur during SSRI treatment. If it becomes very heavy, it may be a sign of fever. Use of the drug should be stopped, and your doctor called.

Tolerating the SSRIs

Nearly every textbook and journal article says that Paxil and the other SSRIs are well tolerated, and therefore ideal for months and years of maintenance therapy to prevent recurrence. I believe it would be more accurate to say the SSRIs are better tolerated than the older tricyclics. Eugene Duboff, M.D., in his article entitled "Long-Term Treatment of Major Depressive Disorder with Paroxetine [Paxil]" in the December 1993 *Journal of Clinical Psychopharmacology*, records that during a one-year trial on Paxil, "adverse events caused approximately 30 percent of patients to withdraw from the study prematurely." The most common reasons cited were fatigue or sleepiness, nausea, headaches, and sweatiness. He goes on to assert that the drug was well tolerated. This does not sound like "well tolerated" to me. In an eight-week double-blind placebo- and Elavil-controlled study of Zoloft in outpatients with major depression by Frederick W. Reimherr et al., reported in the December 1990 *Journal of Clinical Psychiatry*, the dropout rate in all three patient groups was the same, although the reasons cited were different. In the placebo groups, lack of efficacy was the main cause, while in the drug groups, it was side effects (about 20 percent for Elavil and Zoloft). The Zoloft patients had gastrointestinal complaints and sexual dysfunctions, while the Elavil group suffered from more sleepiness and fatigue, constipation, blurred vision, trouble urinating, and dizziness. Although the dropout rate was the same, the Elavil patients had more and worse side effects. In another eight-week double-blind study comparing Zoloft and Elavil in elderly depressed patients, Cal K. Cohn, M.D., et al. reported (also in the December 1990 *Journal of Clinical Psychiatry*) a dropout rate of 28 percent for Zoloft and 35 percent for Elavil. Zoloft won, but hardly overwhelmingly. Without quoting all the other studies and statistics, which make for dull reading, I only wish to sum up by saying that the SSRIs are better tolerated in most studies than Elavil and Tofranil, but their side effects still cause about 20 percent of those taking them to drop out within six weeks, and probably another 10 percent within the first year. There are real advantages to the SSRIs, which I will summarize at the end of this chapter, but they are not perfect, and many people have difficulty tolerating them.

Drug/SSRI Interactions

Since you may be on an SSRI for months, even years, it is important to know how other drugs that you may be taking, or may need to take in the future, will be affected by the SSRIs. Fortunately, the list of serious interactions is not long. Since the SSRIs are metabolized by the liver, they may force up the blood level of a second drug broken down in the same way. If the second drug has a narrow margin between its therapeutic action and toxic level, this can be dangerous. Another source of interaction trouble occurs when two drugs act on the same target. Thus, SSRIs can increase the tremors caused by lithium, and can also produce central serotonin syndrome when combined with MAOIs (which should never be done) and, to a lesser extent, with tryptophan and meperidine (Demerol). This interaction can be especially dangerous when an MAOI is given within six weeks after use of Prozac has been discontinued, since it takes that long for Prozac to be completely cleared from the body.

When tricyclics are combined with SSRIs (in cases where the SSRIs alone are not successful), it must be remembered that less than the normal dose of the tricyclic should be taken, because the SSRI forces the blood level of the tricyclic up two or more times, which could be dangerous if the normal dose were used.

When beginning SSRI treatment, some people become sleepy, and will become more so if they drink alcohol. But those who are not made sleepy by SSRIs can drink their normal amount without any added effect from the drug.

Only MAOIs and tryptophan must be avoided with the SSRIs. The drugs listed below must be used cautiously because of interactions, and under the close supervision of your physician.

Drugs Interacting with All SSRIs
Anticonvulsants
Lithium
Antiarrhythmics
Beta-blockers
Anticoagulants
Antihistamines
Antiulcer drugs
Antianxiety drugs
Phenothiazine antipsychotics
Tricyclic antidepressants

SSRI Dosage

Dosage depends on the individual patient and must be set after careful consultation between you and your physician. In general, if your symptoms are not unbearable, it makes sense to start low and increase the dosage slowly. The following table can be used as a guide.

	Starting Dose (mg)	Daily Dose (mg)
Prozac (fluoxetine)	5–20	20– 80
Zoloft (sertraline)	25–50	100–200
Paxil (paroxetine)	10–20	20– 50
Luvox (fluvoxamine)	50	150–300

Some people can tolerate 20 mg of Prozac from the start, but many feel wired or drugged, or suffer abdominal distress, and do better on 5 or 10 mg. The manufacturer (Eli Lilly) later issued a 10-mg capsule because many people could not take 20 mg right away. Lilly also came out with a liquid form containing 20 mg per teaspoon for those who wish to find out exactly how much they need. From a financial point of view, the 20-mg capsule is cheapest, and the liquid form most expensive. Two 10-mg capsules cost much more than one 20-mg capsule. It may be wise to get a small supply of 10s at first and, once you are comfortable on 20 mg, to shift over. Zoloft comes in scored tablets of 50 and 100 mg, so that it can be divided in half (or less), and the Paxil 20-mg tablet is also scored (it also comes in a 30-mg nonscored version). Luvox comes in 50- and 100-mg scored tablets.

The rate of dosage elevation should be slowest for Prozac, since it builds up in the body over several weeks. For those starting on 20 mg, no dosage elevation should be attempted within the first month, even if there has been little response. Then an increase of 10 mg per month might be tried. Those who are impatient and want to hurry the elevation may pay the price of more side effects, but these are almost always annoying rather than serious, and for those people in a lot of distress, it may be worth it. Prozac is best taken in the morning with food, unless it causes drowsiness, in which case it should be taken after the evening meal.

Zoloft can be taken after the evening meal, as can Paxil, unless it causes agitation or insomnia, in which case it can be taken after breakfast. It can be started with a whole pill or half of one pill, and moved up every week or two until a full response occurs. If after a maximum of several months of 200 mg of Zoloft or 50 mg of Paxil there is still no response, use of the drug should be discontinued. Use of the SSRIs should not be discontinued suddenly, but slowly and gradually.

Luvox can be begun at 50 mg and increased to a maximum of 300 mg. It has been released in the United States only for obsessive compulsive disorder, but has been used worldwide for depression with success.

Much has been made of the fact that Prozac is eliminated from the body only gradually, and some argue that the side effects are much worse because of this. For this reason, many believe that shorter-acting Paxil and Zoloft are more desirable. In my practice, I have not found it to make much difference. When use of Prozac is stopped because of side effects, those effects linger for a month, while those of the other two disappear immediately. If the next drug planned is an MAOI after an SSRI failure, then the wait would only have to be two weeks with Paxil and Zoloft instead of five weeks with Prozac, but that is a theoretical advantage which only rarely comes up.

What's in a Name?

The naming of modern antidepressants is no accident. Clearly, I do not know what went on behind closed doors as the pharmaceutical companies went over what to call these wonder drugs, but here are some of my associations to how they are trying to subliminally influence doctors to prescribe and patients to take these agents.

Prozac. What would have happened if it had been called antizac?

Zoloft. The ball was propelled in a high arc as it was lofted into the outfield; this drug is no strikeout or grounder.

Paxil. From the Latin word *pax*, which means peace, the opposite of anguish.

Wellbutrin. To be well, not ill.

Effexor. To be effective, competent, in charge.

Serzone. To be the Sir, the commander of the zone.

Luvox. In Latin, *vox* means voice, but this name is not satisfactory unless one knows that *luv* means love in old English. In the following section, I will provide detailed explorations of Prozac, Zoloft, Paxil, and Luvox.

Remeron. A *remedy* for depression, or REMeron to restore normal REM sleep.

Prozac (Fluoxetine)

Making the Prozac Decision

As Prozac has become overwhelmingly popular, the matter of who should take it has become muddled. Originally released for the treatment of major depression, its use has spread to many other conditions. Not only are people with eating, sexual, and anxiety disorders, depressives, schizophrenics, obsessive-compulsives, and post-traumatic stress disorder patients candidates for Prozac, but also those who are subsyndromal: the timid; those with low energy and low self-esteem; those who are irritable, perfectionist, inflexible, or suffering from a general malaise or unhappiness; and those who are too aggressive or abusive. In short, anyone—sick or not—may benefit from the civilizing effects of Prozac.

The physician legally controls distribution of the drug through the prescription pad, but since the definition of need (the so-called indication) is broadly (one could say nonexistent), the patient's suffering and wish for the drug often become the deciding factors. Unfortunately, the nature of serotonin is about as clear as that of the id, and its effect on practice may be the same: everyone, no matter what the diagnosis, became a candidate for psychoanalysis or therapy, and now becomes one for Prozac. Six million Americans have taken Prozac. Much of this use is warranted, but clearly some is not. Except in cases of severe major depression, there is no science to guide the physician in the decision to prescribe Prozac. If there is marked interference with your daily functioning, and you are in a lot of pain, then you should persuade your doctor to let you try it for at least several months. The risk of harm is small, and the chance of benefit great.

The Benefits of Prozac

Large, controlled studies of Prozac have established its effectiveness in major depression to be equal to that of the tricyclic antidepressants (e.g., Elavil and Tofranil), with fewer side effects. There are studies of its use in other well-defined conditions which support its prescription in obsessive-compulsive disorder, bulimia, premenstrual dysphoric disorder, and other diagnostic types discussed in the earlier part of this chapter concerning SSRIs in general. With respect to its use in the timid, irritable, overly sensitive, insecure, and fatigued, and those lacking self-confidence, Prozac's success has been established by anecdote rather than controlled study. Anecdotal evidence can be as reliable as the reports of miracles, but that does not make either of them untrue. There are many people who believe Prozac has restored them to full functioning, and I am convinced from my own observation that they are right in their belief. But a large group feel only somewhat better, and others have been hurt by the drug. It is the physician's duty to know what can go wrong and watch for it carefully over time, even if the decision to take Prozac has been handed over to the patient out of the doctor's ignorance, as opposed to carelessness. If a person says to me that he is suffering and I think there is a reasonable chance Prozac will relieve him, I feel obliged to prescribe it. I consider this no more irresponsible than if a postsurgical patient complained of pain and I issued a narcotic. However, I would not prescribe morphine for someone with chronic low-grade back pain, because it is dangerous to do so. The question is, how dangerous is it to prescribe Prozac for more vague, nondisease conditions, ones that are either subsyndromal or perhaps matters of temperament and character rather than syndromes or even subsyndromes?

How Does Prozac Work?

Because the serotonin story remains a mystery, and because no one has proven that depressives have too little of it, it seems more useful to think of Prozac's actions in terms used by those who take it.

In major depression, the reduction in anxiety, bodily aches and pains, trouble thinking and concentrating, sleep distur-bance, motor retardation, and depressed mood has been measured both on the basis of patients' and physicians' accounts of their overall impressions and by means of special-ized depression scales administered by trained raters who did not know if the patient was on a drug or a placebo. The way Prozac works in the large variety of other psychiatric disorders it has been used to treat is, I think, as follows:

As an Anti-Rage Drug

On Prozac, the physically abusive strike out less or not at all, the formerly irritable no longer scream in frustration, and the overly aggressive become less abrasive. Prozac can be thought of as a calming and civilizing drug.

The obvious bad side effect of this is that one can become tranquil in situations in which it would be more appropriate to cry out. One of my patients entered into an abusive inti-mate relationship while on Prozac. When he went off the drug, he realized the relationship had been a terrible mis-take. The doctor and the person considering Prozac must not only identify the presence of anger, rage, and aggression, but evaluate these emotions in the context of the person's life. Are they signals that should be attended to and used as data upon which to form judgments, or are they pathologic aber-rations requiring Prozac for their removal?

Improved Effectiveness

Whether the source of feeling strong and in control comes from the mind actually working better or from improved morale and self-esteem, which bring the expectation of success, the person on Prozac has a sense of being more effective and therefore likely to overcome obstacles. Thus, the person with a history of social phobia is able to give a speech or enter a room of strangers, and someone who never spoke up at sales meetings will begin to do so.

The relationship of anxiety and depression to self-esteem is well known. If your heart is racing with fear and dread of the future, or if you feel stupid and inept because of depression, then you will not expect to overcome the novel and difficult situations you encounter at work or in your social life. Whether your mind functions better, your self-esteem is improved, your anxiety or depression relieved, or your hopes raised—whatever the reason—you feel more in control and effective, and thus your performance improves.

The Pleasure Center Is Turned On

Prozac is not a euphoriant giving people a high like marijuana or cocaine, but like other antidepressants, it turns on the pleasure center that depression extinguishes. A main reason why people feel depressed, lose interest in previously enjoyed activities, stop eating, have no energy, and are unable to concentrate and make decisions is that they anticipate no pleasure from these activities. When Prozac activates the pleasure center, normal appetites and interests return. The depressive's social withdrawal ends; friends are called in the anticipation of a good time. Desire for food and sex returns because they promise enjoyment, and life seems worth sustaining. The pain and misery gone, pleasure once again rewards and motivates activities.

Decreased Sensitivity

Many depressives are thin-skinned and easily hurt by a snub

or an unintended slight. They may agonize for hours after a social gathering about why someone did not speak to or dance with them or what a particular remark meant that seemed to wound them. Some of these sufferers actively seek one social event after another, motivated by a feeling of emptiness and sadness and a desire for relief through human contact, but often they are disappointed by snubs and rejections that less sensitive people would not even have noticed. Like many symptoms of depression, this one is connected to many of the others. If you feel worthless and have low self-esteem, you are much more easily hurt than if you are sure of yourself. If your pleasure center is turned off and you are already in pain, a snub hurts more than if you feel well. The same goes for criticism, which shakes the fragile equilibrium of the depressive, and therefore can be tolerated less well than by the nondepressed.

Prozac makes the depressed person less sensitive to slights and criticism, and more able to consider the suggestions of a boss or family member without overreacting with hurt or rage.

Increased Hope

Depressed people are negative about their abilities, and about the past and the future. Feeling without hope, they are unable to plan their lives, from the smallest social event to the largest project, and are plagued by passivity and indecision. If you ask them to the movies on a Saturday night, they cannot give a straight answer, since they do not know whether they will feel well enough to go. Once again, the symptoms of depression are related to one another. Without the ability to experience pleasure, it is hard to hope that future action will be fruitful. If you feel ineffective and worthless, it is impossible to believe that your efforts will be rewarded, so that you are filled with hopeful anticipation. Without hope, people sit still and alone, unable to motivate themselves to act. Once Prozac restores hope, the person begins to plan social activities, and at work is able to take the many small steps leading to the completion of a big project or sale.

What Is Unique About How Prozac Works?

The five things I have just discussed—decreased rage, increased self-esteem, activation of the pleasure center, diminished sensitivity, and the restoration of hope—are not unique to Prozac. The other SSRIs are all equally capable of producing these results. The older antidepressants certainly could turn on the pleasure center, restore hope, and increase self-esteem, but because of their tricky dose schedules (from one to twelve pills) and their annoying side effects (dry mouth, constipation, blood pressure drop, racing pulse, weight gain, blurred vision), their use was reserved for more severe depressions, and given in ineffective, inadequate dosages by nonspecialists. Thus, the large group of nonmajor depressives—the shy, the overly sensitive, the obsessed, the impulsive, the insecure, the irritable, and the aggressive— were rarely if ever medicated using the older antidepressants, and almost never in adequate dosages because the side effects would have made them intolerable.

In the general population, rage, along with physical and verbal abuse, nasty impatience, and a hostile confrontational attitude, are diminished by the SSRIs, as they never were before by the older antidepressants. Hypersensitivity to rejection and criticism, fearfulness, timidity, shyness, rigidity, perfectionism, and impulsivity are all affected by Prozac and the other SSRIs.

Prozac is not different from the other SSRIs, it was simply there first, used most, and has been the focus of the largest mythology. Zoloft, Paxil, and Luvox have never appeared on the covers of popular magazines, or been singled out for attack by the Scientologists. Prozac is the name everybody knows, the one appearing on book titles. It is the drug people are likely to ask for.

Prozac Is Middle-Aged

In early 1997, Prozac will have been available for nine years in the United States. Many of the hottest controversies about it have been settled, and it is rarely seen on magazine covers these days. Many who have tried it have now stopped taking it, because it worked and they feel better, because they did not like the way it made them feel, or because it did not do much for them. Some who come to my office have tried it and want something new.

New drugs are like new lovers. First, there is the excitement of finding out about the promise of unknown benefits, accompanied by nervousness about undiscovered dangers. After a while, the pluses and minuses surface, resulting in a comfortable status quo or the decision to move on to someone or something better. Among the SSRIs and other newly available antidepressants, no one drug stands out as the best. They offer seductive alternatives, especially to those disappointed by Prozac. The attractions of the other anti-depressants will be described in the sections in which they are considered, but some of these are siren songs with known and hidden dangers. Where possible, the use of older drugs whose characteristics are understood is safer and preferable to use of the latest one, whose harms are unknown.

Women and Prozac

As I begin to tell you about seven of the hundreds of people I have significantly helped with Prozac, I notice that five are women—slightly over 70 percent. Since most studies find that women make up 67 percent of those suffering from depressions, my 70 percent could simply reflect the national average. But many of the people I am about to describe are not major depressives. Rather, the fact that there is a preponderance of women reflects something else I have found in my clinical practice. Women are more willing to accept help when they need it, and do not have to be in the driver's seat or hold the TV remote control. Taking a psychiatric drug for depression or other mental condition is perceived by most people to be different from talking therapy, and to imply that the condition is more serious, that they cannot handle it by themselves and need medication. Many men resist this need, seeing it as a sign of weakness and a form of dependence. Women, perhaps more realistic and practical, are more willing to accept the necessary and to be open to advice from an expert. Men find it more threatening when they are ill and needy, subject to forces they cannot completely control. Since all human beings are subject to illness and forces beyond their control, perhaps men are the weaker sex in light of their reluctance to recognize and accept this state of nature.

Seven Prozac Success Stories

Although I am about to briefly tell you about seven Prozac successes, I must remind you that Prozac cures only about 30 percent of the severely depressed, and about 70 percent of all the depressed. It has done a lot of good, and continues to do so, but it is not a miracle drug. I include seven successes simply to show what it does when it works.

Out of Bed

Thirty-two-year-old Barbara needed to feel up and confident to go out on sales calls. Instead, she languished in bed and was in no condition to sell herself or her products. After two months of Prozac, she was not only back selling successfully but making plans for her future.

Tears and No Man

A thirty-six-year-old stranger in a new city, Laura burst into tears at work, and felt lonely, less capable than the other middle managers, and unable to attract a suitable man. Prozac steadily raised her level of confidence and stopped her tears. Feeling better for six months, she decided to stop taking the drug, but her improvement continued. Performing well at work, she was promoted. She fell in love and has plans to marry.

No Longer Punching His Wife

Twenty-seven-year-old Jim would periodically punch and hurt his wife, but never touched the children. He denied being depressed or even angry with his wife, and said the blows (he sometimes hurt his fist punching the wall) were delivered impulsively, unexpectedly, and without reason. I made the diagnosis of intermittent explosive disorder and prescribed Prozac. The punches stopped.

The Ability and Courage to Speak Out

At the age of twenty-six, Eliza had just gotten a promotion that required her to make presentations to the senior management of her company, a prospect which terrified her: she was certain she would do badly. In addition, she was reluctant to speak up in other situations, even among her friends, because she believed her thoughts to be dull. She had long periods of social withdrawal accompanied by feelings of boredom, sadness, and low self-esteem. I made the diagnosis of dysthymia and started her on Prozac. Several weeks later, she felt vastly improved. Not only did she have the courage to speak up at senior management meetings, she was convinced her mind worked better.

Eliza not only felt more confident, her mind actually began to function better. One important factor in depression is its effect on thinking. The minds of depressed people are slowed; they experience a poverty of thoughts, their concentration is faulty, and in elderly people, depression can produce a false dementia with disorientation and impaired memory, judgment, and intellect. Eliza is not a dramatic person whose speech is filled with exaggeration. When she said her thoughts were more lucid, evolved, and complete when she was on Prozac, I tended to believe her.

Less Angry and Critical

Frank was fifty-five years old, worked hard as a college administrator, and came home tired and intolerant. He expected his wife to wait on him and to attend to the home, which was his oasis. She worked hard at her job, too, and wished to retire from her post as Frank's servant. Her failure to care for him properly enraged Frank, who looked daggers at her but said little. Instead, he poured himself a few too many stiff drinks, and sometimes these disinhibited him, and out poured vicious remarks toward his wife. These she attributed to the effects of alcohol rather than to the need for adjustments and compromises in their marriage. The diagnosis in this case was episodic alcoholism and marital relational problems. After several weeks on Prozac, Frank felt less inclined to drink and appeared less angry toward his wife. The angry look on his face had mostly disappeared.

Frank's case was not a Prozac cure. He continued to drink occasionally and to feel angry toward his wife. The value of the drug lay in the fact that he was more able to articulate his displeasure instead of silently raging or intermittently exploding aided by alcohol. The work with his psychotherapist was aided, not superseded, by the drug.

I'll Never Have a Family

Barbara was thirty-five, unmarried, anxious, and depressed that she would never marry or have a family. Her superior intelligence, good looks, and attractive personality made her a success at work, but she remained miserable about her personal life, and was in therapy for several years with little success. Diagnostically, she was either a dysthymic (chronic mild depression) with an obsession about marriage and children, or a person with an obsessive-compulsive disorder who could not stop thinking about having a family; or perhaps she suffered from a mixed anxiety and depressive syndrome, and felt hopeless and worried about the future. Prozac brought her complete relief, no matter what the correct diagnosis. Those who see the drug as balancing the serotonin system do not worry so much about diagnostic distinctions. She ceased to be convinced of her inability to get what she wanted, and less obsessed, frantic, and depressed, she relaxed and started to achieve her goals. She found a man she loved and felt comfortable with, and began to hope that everything would work out and they would marry.

My Husband Is a Complete Egotist

Evelyn was forty-five and had been married for six years to a man she found selfish, miserly, and childish. She held herself back until she could no longer contain herself, and then complained bitterly to him. He responded by avoiding her, and she ended up feeling worse. Evelyn regarded her situation as hopeless and was considering divorce, but she worried about supporting herself and being alone. Diagnostically, she was hard to classify. She was unhappy but not a depressive; she functioned well at home and at work; and her main symptom was her marriage. She wanted to try Prozac to see if it would alleviate her unhappiness and calm her rage at her husband. This was the kind of situation that I found difficult. There was no clear psychiatric illness; Evelyn did not even have a subsyndromal illness. As a clinician, I felt vulnerable to the charge that I was a pill-pusher, a psychiatric protector of the status quo (Evelyn's marriage), the kind of doctor who drugged women so they would overlook or not respond to mistreatment at the hands of men—in this case, Evelyn's husband.

Two considerations made me go ahead with Prozac. The first rule of medicine is "do no harm." The harm to this woman, whom I had seen for months in psychotherapy and had been unable to help, was to leave her in unnecessary pain. Second, doctors often have to act without a complete diagnosis. When all diagnostic explorations fail, the surgeon may be forced to open the abdomen for exploratory purposes. The orthopedist, unable to discover the source of back pain, may prescribe medication, a change in diet, and exercise. The allergist, unable to find the reason for red and itchy eyes, may offer drops. I had a patient in pain and no diagnosis, and decided to proceed. This may seem irresponsible to the ethicist, but necessary to the clinician with a patient in pain.

Prozac produced a curious result in Evelyn. She was able to hold back her sharp, impulsive retorts at her childish, selfish husband, and to consider what effect her words might have on him, and how best to get him to do what she wanted. She decided she would get much further with her egoist if she flattered him and seemed grateful for all he had done for her. It worked like a charm. He began to come home earlier, and even offered to help by doing the dishes. Her marriage became much happier. Furthermore, she was able to observe this sequence of events and learn from it. The idea that one either gains insight in psychotherapy or is cured by Prozac is a false dichotomy set up by those involved in a debate. When emotions are in control, people can learn for themselves through experience or with the help of a therapist.

Can Prozac Make People Worse?

Prozac can make someone worse if that person becomes manic, paranoid, has a seizure, develops a skin rash, or has a bad interaction with another drug. These dangers have been covered in the preceding section on SSRIs. The notion that Prozac induces suicide has been disproved. Dr. Martin Teicher, the author of the report that came to the conclusion that the drug could lead to suicide, recently told me that his findings were incorrect. Unfortunately, once something is in the medical literature, it is hard to get it out.

It is in the area of personality and temperament that the most interesting changes for the worse occur. It is a rule of medicine that every treatment which has an effect also produces a side effect. Thus, if the meek can be empowered, they can be made too much so, while the assertive can become lacking in sensitivity and tact, excessively forward and brash. If the irritable and rageful can be calmed, then they can be made too meek, while the normally assertive may become too forgiving.

Finally, there is the problem of the incomplete cure. If the psychiatrist monitors the patient for side effects, it is also necessary to carefully watch for the partial failure to recover, for in this category lies much misery and loss of capacity to function. Partially recovered depressives suffer largely unrecognized and unhelped by their physicians.

The following are three cases illustrating Prozac failures, in the meek, the rageful, and in the depressed:

Frank

Forty-nine-year-old Frank had been a machinist until several years ago when he decided to try to become an engineer. He took courses and tests qualifying him to assume this role. During his long, bitter divorce, he suffered a major depressive episode. He was put on Prozac, and it sped his recovery. He decided to remain on it while he interviewed for a new job.

It was during his description of an interview that I realized that this normally sensitive and cautious man was being harmed by Prozac. He felt the interviewer was trying to trick him in order to test him. Normally Frank would have noticed this and handled himself and the interviewer skillfully. Instead he said, "I'm not going to fall for that one," and openly discussed the trap he felt was being set. The interviewer said nothing, but I was not surprised when Frank was turned down.

Frank could be labeled either hypomanic due to Prozac, or a previously undiagnosed bipolar, whose brashness was due to pressure of speech and grandiosity, and his desire to become an engineer inspired by an elevated mood. But his mood was not "clearly different" from his normal one, and if his ambition to improve himself were grandiosity, then everyone seeking a job promotion must be sick. His thoughts were not racing; he was not distractible, agitated, sleepless, involved in buying sprees, sexual indiscretions, or foolish investments. I did not think him hypomanic. What I did think was that

Frank had been tipped by Prozac from being sensitive to being insensitive, from considering the consequences of his behavior to being oblivious, and from being normally cautious to being impulsive.

Barbara

Forty-one-year-old Barbara divorced after ten years of marriage. She became accustomed to living alone and enjoyed her job. But she was given to outbursts of temper, and this, plus her chronic boredom and dissatisfaction, led to her being placed on Prozac. As a consequence, her relationships with her brothers, sisters, and parents vastly improved. She tolerated their faults much better, and stopped hanging up phones and walking angrily out of rooms. She was very grateful for Prozac's calming effect on her previously tempestuous family ties. Unfortunately, the Prozac effect went too far.

Barbara met an unemployed woman, became friendly, and let her move in. She supported her, let her use the car, and did whatever she asked. Her new roommate would criticize and ridicule Barbara virtually nonstop, stay out overnight without notice or explanation, and refuse to keep her company on weekends. Finally, after a year of verbal abuse and inconsiderate behavior, Barbara asked her to leave. Several months later, when off Prozac, she described how the drug not only had calmed her rages but had made her too tranquil, willing to tolerate her former roommate's freeloading and harassment, something she would never have permitted when off the drug.

Joyce

Joyce was forty-seven years old, married, with three children. She had been chronically depressed for over twenty years, the last six of which she had been on 20 to 60 mg of Prozac, depending upon the severity of her chronically moderate depression. When it was at its worst, psychotic thoughts entered her mind, and she began to feel the neighbors were talking about her and saying uncomplimentary things.

If we measured Joyce's condition using the Hamilton Depression Scale (see p. 36), Joyce would be considered improved, perhaps even cured, after taking Prozac. But only one of the seventeen items on the scale involves work and interests, which means one could be scored as nondepressed, yet not work or have any interests. I believe that almost all drug studies contain this weakness in the Hamilton scale, one that is slowly being recognized by researchers interested in social adjustment and quality of life following depression.

Social Adjustment After Prozac

Prozac moves most people in the right direction, but it is very important to think about where you are starting from. If you are severely depressed, it will take longer for you to respond than if you are mildly ill. Prozac successes among the timid, irritable, fatigued, abusive, and insecure who do not have major depression are gratifying for doctor and patient. Giovanni Cassano et al. studied social adjustment in 176 patients with mild to moderate depression. They found that those on tricyclic antidepressants who reported improvement were able to work and felt well, but their relationships with spouses and children remained impaired, and they participated in few leisure and social activities. These researchers suggested that impairment in the capacity to enjoy leisure may remain constant during some depressed people's lifetimes. I have seen this happen with certain chronically depressed people on Prozac, too. Some recover their leisure and social interests very slowly, long after the rest of their depressed symptoms have disappeared. Others, unfortunately, are able to work and carry out the tasks necessary in their lives but have no hobbies, interests, or passions. These are the loners, the workaholics, and the idle shut-ins. This is the main reason why most depressives need more than drugs to be truly cured. They need help getting along with their spouses, children, neighbors, and friends, and in finding activities that will give them pleasure.

Dr. William Coryell et al. studied 148 bipolar and 240 unipolar affective disorder patients at the time they sought treatment and again five years later, and compared their overall functioning to that of their nondepressed relatives. In their report, Dr. Coryell and his colleagues noted the "enduring psychosocial consequences of mania and depression" and found that five years after the onset of illness, the depressed were less likely to be employed and to have been promoted at work, and more likely to have lower incomes. In addition, unipolar and bipolar patients were only half as likely to have ever been married, and those married were twice as often divorced or separated. The unipolars who remained married were unhappy both with their marriage and with their sex lives. Dr. Coryell's group found the impairment of seemingly recovered depressives to remain serious: their job status and incomes continued to decline; their marriages were still miserable, and their sexual relationships unhappy. The authors note that their sample of depressed subjects may have been sicker on average, and thus more chronically impaired, for they were recruited from five specialized care centers. They question the usual practice of defining recovery from depression in terms of an absence of symptoms, while overlooking profound psychosocial damage. While the detriment may grow less the longer the person is symptom-free, these authors believe impairment to be life-long in many cases.

We need more studies of the effects of major depression on marriage, work, and leisure-time activities. While many people recover fully, many others require much more than the symptomatic relief provided by Prozac. They need help with their jobs, marriages, sexual functioning, friendships, and with their leisure-time activities. Work and pleasure must also improve, not just the other sixteen items on the Hamilton Depression Scale.

Prozac's Interactions with Other Drugs

Although I have discussed this subject generally in the section on SSRIs, I wish to bring it up again here with respect to Prozac for two reasons. It is the subject of intense interest and recent research, and because Prozac lingers in the body for weeks, it affects not only those drugs you already are on but those you may take in the future. Thus, five weeks must elapse after you stop taking Prozac before you can start the MAOIs, Nardil, or Parnate. While MAOIs, L-tryptophan, and the anti–Parkinson's disease drug L-deprenyl (Eldepryl) must *never* be taken along with Prozac, other drugs can and will be, but it is necessary to know how they will be affected. For example, the effect of the tricyclic antidepressant desipramine will be increased many times by Prozac. Thus, when combined with Prozac, desipramine must be used in a lower than normal dosage. To a lesser extent, Prozac magnifies the effect of Valium and Xanax. Prozac also increases the effect of Clozaril, and therefore the risk of seizure associated with the latter.

The effect of Prozac on these other drugs is mediated through Prozac's effect on liver metabolism. No one knows whether long-term use of Prozac will harm the liver. Up to now, however, Prozac does not seem especially toxic to the liver.

Taking Prozac for the Rest of Your Life

There are two types of major depressives: those people who suffer only from depression, and those who suffer from mania and depression. The first typically have four to six episodes in their lifetime; the bipolars, seven to nine periods of acute illness. Furthermore, unipolar episodes occur closer together and become more severe and long-lasting as the person gets older. One study at the University of Pittsburgh found that half of unipolar and bipolar depressives who stop taking their medication relapse in one year. Furthermore, the older a person is when suffering a first episode, the more likely there will be a recurrence in two years. Therefore, I would advise severe major depressives who have had three episodes, those over age forty who have had two episodes, and those over age fifty who have had one episode, to remain on an SSRI for life. Another reason for long-term Prozac use is the presence of residual symptoms following an acute episode or the presence of incapacitating dysthymia. I realize that taking Prozac continuously carries unknown risks, which I hope will not be serious, but severe major depressive disorder is also serious, recurs, and requires continuous medication for its prevention.

As for those taking Prozac for milder but nonetheless painful and limiting emotional states, I would suggest trying to come off the medication after a year or two. Although whatever it was that made you start taking Prozac may come back, the symptom-free period in between may have helped you acquire new social and stress-reducing skills, either with or without a psychotherapist, and you may find that you no longer need Prozac. If this is not the case, go back on it, but with the intention of doing so for a limited time only. I have seen many people outgrow their need for Prozac. Only the severe major depressive needs it for life.

When discontinuing use of Prozac, do so gradually. If you are on more than one capsule, reduce it by one every few weeks. Once you are down to one capsule a day, start to space it out to every other, and then every third, day. The reason for this is that if you stop taking the drug suddenly, you may become anxious or depressed, or feel unwell and mistake this for proof that you still need Prozac. In fact, what you are experiencing is a withdrawal reaction. I used to think that because Prozac lasts for weeks in the system, gradual withdrawal should be unnecessary, but I have seen people develop unpleasant symptoms from the sudden withdrawal of the drug.

Prozac and Severe PMS (Premenstrual Syndrome)

The *American Psychiatric Press Textbook of Psychiatry* (2d ed., 1994) notes that "both men and women attribute negative psychological states and behaviors in women to the menstrual cycle" and laments the lack of good diagnostic criteria and treatment for this condition. Thus, there is great controversy surrounding the use of Prozac for treating premenstrual syndrome.

Dr. Barbara Parry, a professor of psychiatry at the University of California at San Diego, writes that in PMS "the mood and behavioral changes are recurrent and predictable." These changes can be divided into mood and bodily complaints. The mood changes include depression, fatigue, anxiety, tension, irritability, and headache. The bodily changes include abdominal bloating, breast tenderness, and ankle swelling. Dr. Parry reviews a long list of mostly unsatisfactory attempts to treat PMS. Open trials of various drugs initially look promising, only to prove ineffective when subjected to controlled, double-blind review.

One double-blind study of PMS by Dr. Andrea Stone (1991) found Prozac to be effective in treating both the mood and physical symptoms associated with PMS. But even in this carefully designed study, which by its rigor was able to eliminate placebo responders, 50 percent had a history of major depression. Nonetheless, women whose PMS was sufficiently severe as to seriously interfere with their social or occupational functioning were helped. A larger, but less rigorous, double-blind study reported by Dr. Meir Steiner in the *New England Journal of Medicine* (June 8, 1995) also found Prozac to be more effective than a placebo.

Who Should Start on Less Than 20 mg of Prozac a Day?

In 1988, when Prozac was released in the United States, only 20-mg capsules were available, forcing many on the drug to open the capsules, pour the contents into cranberry juice, leave the mixture in the refrigerator, and drink half one day and half the next. After complaints and several years of "cranzac," the 10-mg capsule and the liquid form were released. The existence of only a 20-mg capsule initially had an important positive effect, in that it forced people to be on a full therapeutic dose from the start. In spite of subsequent refinements, there seems to be something almost magical about the 20-mg dose, and debate continues among experts who think a dose of 40 to 80 mg makes more people better than does 20 mg, and those who find no advantage—the so-called flat dose response curve. Since many who received the older tricyclics were on too low a dosage, Prozac helped many more people because it was given in adequate amounts.

There are three kinds of people who should start on less than 20 mg a day. First, those who suffer panic attacks or who are very anxious in general, who may find the SSRI side effects of nervousness, insomnia, and anxiety intolerable. A lower dosage (5 mg) allows you to become accustomed to the drug gradually, and then the dosage can be raised. The other two kinds of people who should be started on less than 20 mg are the elderly, who metabolize and excrete the drug more slowly, and those with liver or kidney disease. Prozac is effective in the elderly, although no more so than any other SSRI, and causes fewer side effects than the tricyclics. It increases the blood levels of other antidepressants, which should therefore be used in lower than normal dosages.

If you elect to begin Prozac at 10 mg or less, and are in good medical health, and if you are not bothered by side effects, then it is wise to increase the dose to 20 mg after a week. Although some people may not need this, most do, and it will speed the response. Depression is painful, and the sooner gone, the better. There is a small percentage (under 10 percent) who metabolize Prozac slowly, and they may require lower dosage.

106 PROZAC AND THE NEW ANTIDEPRESSANTS

Double Depression and Prozac

Chronic depression of varying severity punctuated by episodes of acute major depression is called double depression. This concept is important because it used to be thought that acute major depression was self-limited and followed by complete recovery, and now it is known that about 20 percent do not recover completely. These people are candidates for continuous Prozac treatment, which not only shortens and diminishes the intensity of the acute episode but also can relieve the impairment associated with chronic double depression.

Childhood and Adolescent Depression and Prozac

Since 1950, there has been an increased rate of depression in children and adolescents. Major depression in young people is a chronic and recurring condition, so that 40 percent suffer a second depressive episode within two years, and 70 percent in five years. These children and adolescents are affected in their school performance and in their relationships with peers and family. They are also likely to have conduct disorders and conflicts with their mothers and fathers. The condition persists into adulthood and continues to affect their work, social, and family life. There is a high risk of suicide in the young depressed group.

Despite several attempts at placebo-controlled studies of antidepressants in child and adolescent depression, no difference has been found between the effects of the drug and those of the placebo. Unfortunately, no psychotherapy or drug therapy of early-onset depression has been effective in unipolar or bipolar children or adolescents. Nonetheless, Prozac and other antidepressants are widely used in depressed young people by clinicians who believe them to be effective. There is no general consensus as to which children are most likely to benefit at what dose and how long they should be treated. Children and adolescents do respond well to Prozac; it is just that they respond well to a placebo, too, and it is this high placebo response rate that makes it so difficult to establish Prozac's superiority over a sugar pill. Since childhood and adolescent depression often progresses into adult depression, it may just be that when young these individuals are more influenced by the promise of any pill. However, in severe childhood and adolescent depression, neither Prozac nor a placebo seems to do much good.

At this time, the study of depression at both ends of the age spectrum, the young and the old, is intense. We need more answers in both areas. I hope they will come soon. Until then, Prozac is worth a try, but produces no miracles.

Prozac in Acute Bipolar Depression

The danger of antidepressant drug use in bipolar patients is mood destabilization with hypomania or rapid cycling (four or more episodes of mania or depression in a twelve-month period) or both. Thus, once the depression is relieved, the antidepressant is withdrawn, and the mood-stabilizing drug continued alone. Because Prozac has a very long stay in the body, so that the blood level declines by only a half in one month, it may make sense to use a shorter-acting SSRI in bipolar people in case hypomania occurs. Whether antidepressants actually induce mania in bipolar patients or the manic phase is a product of the disease itself (and not drug-caused) has never been adequately researched, and most likely will never be because it would be necessary to deny treatment to half of the depressed bipolar patients, who would be on a placebo.

Prozac in Atypical Depression

The atypical depressive eats and sleeps too much, and is irritable, agitated, oversensitive to rejection, and unresponsive to gladdening events. The oversensitivity to rejection arises in youth and remains throughout most of adult life. It is present both when the person is and is not depressed. Those who are oversensitive to rejection cannot stand criticism at work or from friends and family. Younger people are more likely to exhibit atypical features. Oversensitivity to rejection can interfere with long-term relationships, making them stormy or totally disrupting them, and those so afflicted may avoid intimacy out of fear of being hurt. It also interferes with their relationships with supervisors and others at work.

Studies have repeatedly shown that atypical depressives respond better to the MAOIs Nardil and Parnate than they do to the tricyclic antidepressants Elavil and Tofranil. One recent report found SSRIs to be as effective as MAOIs.

Claire is an example of someone with atypical depression. She is forty-three and is getting divorced after ten years of a stormy marriage. She spent most of those years in therapy complaining about her husband's insensitivity and how it hurt her. She has many women friends and goes to one with tales of mistreatment at the hands of the other. Claire spends hours thinking about what an acquaintance said or did, about a party she went to or to which she was not invited. She prides herself on being sensitive. In fact, she suffers a lot and is oversensitive. At a time when she was depressed and furious with her best friend, she agreed to try Prozac. After several weeks, she began to feel better; her mind was no longer preoccupied with the snubs and wounds she suffered. She became more productive at work and more content with the people in her life.

Prozac and Melancholia

Melancholia is a severe form of depression in which the person experiences complete loss of pleasure and is not cheered up even when something good happens. The melancholic's mood is distinctly different from normal sadness, such as that resulting from the death of a loved one. The depressed mood is worse in the morning; the sufferer wakes up at 2 to

4 A.M. unable to return to sleep, is agitated or slowed, loses a lot of weight, has no appetite, and feels excessive guilt. Melancholics may need hospitalization, and their recovery with antidepressant medication is slow, requiring weeks or months. There is debate over whether the older tricyclic antidepressants are more effective than the SSRIs in treating melancholia, and more studies will be needed to settle it.

Prozac and Euphoria

Euphoria is a feeling of great happiness or well-being, and derives from the Greek word *euphoros*, relating to good health. Prozac is not listed as a cause of euphoria in the American Psychiatric Association's textbook (1994), while alcohol, cocaine, and methadone-induced euphoria are. In the *Physicians' Desk Reference (PDR)*, euphoria is described as occurring infrequently (1 in 100 to 1 in 1,000) among those on Prozac. Dr. Lars F. Gram, in a review of Prozac in the *New England Journal of Medicine* (November 17, 1994), ends by saying, "The published data on the antidepressant effect of fluoxetine [Prozac] do not fully explain its popularity. One may speculate that fluoxetine has psychobiologic effects not strictly related to the biology of depression and that it acts primarily as a mood-or-affect-modulating agent." Does this mean euphoria, and if so, is this good or bad? If one has enthusiasm for a subject or a cause, feels great excitement and interest, is one manic or to be envied? If you have lost all interest in things and are suffering from a melancholic depression, should euphoria be viewed as a return of health or a sickness? Do you really feel great interest and excitement in what you are doing or are you merely high from a pill? Are you in love or the victim of a love potion? The line between feeling well and being slightly manic can be unclear.

The *Diagnostic and Statistical Manual* (4th ed., 1994; *DSM IV*) describes the elevated mood characteristic of a manic episode as "euphoric, unusually good, cheerful, or high . . . [and] it is recognized as excessive by those who know the person well." It then goes on to describe the enthusiasm as "indiscriminate" and the accompanying self-esteem as "inflated," even grandiose. The mood, according to the *DSM IV* must be abnormally elevated for at least a week. I will not repeat here the earlier sections on manic and hypomanic episodes, but will only say that Prozac, in my experience, induces what I would call a "healthy" euphoria or feeling of confidence, well-being, and enthusiasm in a significant percentage of the people I treat with it, and in a small minority an excessive high, one in which their loved ones find them abnormally excited by routine events. This latter hypomanic group presents a diagnostic problem if they live alone and are not sufficiently intimate with anyone for their excitement about the routine to be called to their (or a physician's) attention, because they run the risk of unintentionally alienating coworkers and customers with their brash and insensitive behavior. When an individual becomes clinically manic, it is easy for strangers to spot; the hypomanic's expansive or irritable mood, distractibility, excessive activity, and talkativeness may be more difficult for others to distinguish as abnormal. It is this latter continuum from healthy euphoria to mild hypomania that the individual who crosses that line will not notice for himself, and he will end up suffering the social and occupational consequences. Hypomanics can be energetic, cheerful, productive, and enjoyable to be around, but they can also be disorganized, distractible, irritable, and lacking in social judgment—attributes into which they have no insight and which can get them in trouble at home and on the job. When I noted earlier that Prozac is not a euphoriant, I should have added a qualifier. I should have said that Prozac is often a healthy euphoriant and only occasionally causes loss of judgment and abnormal euphoria (hypomania).

"Me, Too" Drugs

Eli Lilly and Co.'s 1996 Prozac sales are predicted at $2.3 billion, leading other drug companies to market new entries in the SSRI class. A "me, too" drug is a similar product that competes for the same group of patients. The companies then promote the drugs aggressively in an attempt to distinguish their own, even though they can, in fact, barely be told apart. These efforts are aimed at physicians, pharmacists, and sometimes directly at the public. Because Prozac has been such a phenomenal success since 1988, Zoloft (1992), Paxil (1993), and Luvox (1995) have followed. If any of these were to take away even 10 percent of the Prozac share, it would mean $150 million in sales. There are some advantages to the availability of "me, too" drugs. If a person is allergic to one, the presence of a second SSRI in the form of a different chemical compound to which he is not allergic is an advantage. If the side effects are slightly different, one SSRI may be tolerated, while another is not. Since 15 to 20 percent of people discontinue use of their first SSRI because of side effects and another 20 percent stop because they are not being helped, it is useful to have an alternative available.

In spite of a mythology regarding how SSRIs differ, here is a list of their basic similarities:

- All of the SSRIs are equally effective.
- All can be taken once a day.
- One pill daily is usually enough. (Thus, an effective dose can be used from the beginning of treatment.)
- All require days to weeks before they begin to work.
- All prevent relapse equally well.
- An overdose of any of the SSRIs does not affect the heart.
- Their side effects are much more alike than different. What few differences there are will be discussed under each drug.

Since no SSRI is more effective or better tolerated than Prozac, manufacturers have emphasized differences in duration of action, metabolism, age effect, ease in altering blood level, and reduced risk of drug interactions as selling points. Because Prozac and its active metabolite are only half gone in two weeks, whereas Zoloft and Paxil half disappear in one day, all kinds of sinister things can be imagined about Prozac. It can drive mania and interact with MAOIs. So, of course, can the other two, but maybe less so. Unfortunately, the advantage of Zoloft and Paxil in mania is unproven and the need to wait two weeks, versus five weeks for Prozac, before beginning an MAOI rarely comes up. Prozac dosage is harder to adjust than the other two, but this is a theoretical and rarely a clinical problem. When doubt arises about what is a drug side effect (e.g., headache, lethargy), the answer lies in the clinical decision either to maintain the dose to see if the side effect goes away, or to cut the amount. The solution to the problem is no more instantly clear with Zoloft than with Prozac.

The disadvantages of a longer-acting drug are emphasized by those advocating Zoloft, but actually it is the fears of it that rule. The advantages of Prozac are that people may forget to take their drug one day, or fail to fill their prescription. Prozac remains in the body, while Zoloft does not. Also, there needs to be research into whether taking Prozac once or twice a week might not be effective, cheaper, and more convenient.

Zoloft

The sales of Pfizer's Zoloft rose more than 50 percent in 1994 and an additional 38 percent in 1995, and the drug now has one third of the $3 billion modern antidepressant U.S. drug market compared to Prozac's 44 percent. Two leading psychiatric professors, Frederick Goodwin and Sheldon Preskorn, call it the SSRI of choice because one half is excreted by the body in one day (Prozac takes one to two weeks), and because of its lesser effect on liver enzymes. The latter means that Zoloft does not slow its own metabolism when the dose of it is raised, whereas Prozac does, causing its level in the body to increase in a nonlinear fashion. Instead of four pills resulting in a blood level four times higher than with Zoloft, the effect in Prozac capsules is a more than four-fold blood level increase. In addition, the combination of Zoloft with other drugs is more predictable because of its lesser effect on the liver's metabolism of these other drugs. Thus, when desipramine, another antidepressant that may be combined with an SSRI in treatment-resistant patients, is given with Prozac, the former reaches a blood level four times as high as it would have if taken by itself. The same is true when desipramine is combined with Paxil. The combination of Zoloft with desipramine only raises the latter by 40 percent instead of 400 percent, although when doses greater than 50 mg (100 to 200 mg) are used, Zoloft's advantage diminishes.

In my opinion, these fine points of metabolism are of little concern to the overwhelming majority of people who take only Prozac or Zoloft alone and have no need of combining it with other drugs or increasing the dosage. Furthermore, I am concerned about a middle-aged drug like Prozac, whose faults are known, being pushed out by a younger one whose dangers we know less well and that has no particular advantage in terms of its efficacy or side effect profile. After all, desipramine can be used with Prozac if the dose is kept low, and the MAOIs cannot be used with any of the SSRIs. It is not that I am conservative just for its own sake. I was among the first to prescribe Prozac because it had a clear advantage over the drugs that came before it. Zoloft does not. There is an old rule for psychopharmacologists that they should use one drug from each class and know it well. Indeed, it is to the advantage of those for whom they prescribe that they know each drug they prescribe well. This can sometimes mean resisting the latest "me, too" drug. I am still concerned enough about the possible long-term ill effects of Prozac without spreading my concern (and ignorance) to the seven other SSRIs. I tend to reserve the use of Zoloft for occasions when Prozac does not work.

How Does Zoloft Work?

Zoloft reaches maximum concentration in the blood five to eight hours after being ingested, a process aided if the patient takes the drug with food. Whenever a person starts a new intermediate- to long-acting drug, the blood level rises over days to weeks until such time as a so-called steady state occurs, in which the concentration of the drug in the body remains on a plateau, an equilibrium between the daily dose ingested and bodily excretion of the medication. Because it is metabolized faster than Prozac, a steady concentration of Zoloft is reached in the body in one week rather than two to eight weeks. If a second pill must be added because of a failure to respond, the blood level of Zoloft adjusts within one week. This point regarding the speed of blood level adjustment is made much of by Zoloft advocates, although I fail to see the value of it. No one has claimed that Zoloft cures the patient faster or even that the blood levels of SSRIs have any connection to the number of patients who respond. Perhaps there is some advantage to Zoloft's being 97 percent cleared from the body one week after the patient stops taking the drug, whereas Prozac is only half gone in over two weeks, but even here, this is counterbalanced by the disadvantage of having to taper off the Zoloft dose more carefully to avoid withdrawal reactions.

Most SSRI research has been done on outpatients, and thus there has been concern about whether these drugs are as effective as the tricyclics in severe, inpatient depressives. In a large controlled Danish study, severely depressed inpatients responded better to a tricyclic (clomipramine) in comparison to the SSRIs Paxil and Citalopram (not available in the United States). The new serotonin and norepinephrine re-uptake inhibitor Effexor (released in 1994) was found to be superior to Prozac in two studies of severely depressed patients. More research on the SSRIs' effectiveness in depressed inpatients is necessary, but their equal efficacy to tricyclics in outpatients has been established.

SSRIs cause the side effects of agitation, anxiety, and insomnia. Thus, there is concern about how people with a mixture of anxiety and depression or those with recurrent insomnia will be affected. Zoloft has been effective in both the anxious and the sleepless. Neither the severity nor the chronicity of depression diminished the effectiveness of Zoloft, which can be given over a lifetime where necessary.

Dosage

Most people begin taking Zoloft at 50 mg once daily, either in the morning or in the evening. The therapeutic effect is apparent within two to four weeks, as it is with other anti-depressants. After a month, if there is little response, the dose is raised by 50 mg per week until a maximum of 200 mg daily is reached. People with liver or kidney disease or those who are elderly take lower amounts.

Side Effects

As with Prozac, Zoloft can cause headaches, nausea, diar-rhea, insomnia, hand tremors, agitation, and anxiety. Like Prozac, it has little effect on the heart, and thus is much safer than tricyclics in overdosage. Since the threat of suicide always exists in depression, the safety of the SSRIs with respect to possible overdose is particularly important. Zoloft causes less dry mouth, drowsiness, fatigue, dizziness, constipation, and weight gain than the tricyclics.

Efforts to distinguish Zoloft from Prozac on the basis of side effects have not been very successful, as the two drugs are more alike than different. All the SSRIs produce similar sexual dysfunction. Side effects of all the SSRIs are dose-related, so that it makes sense to take the least amount required for a good clinical response. Since it takes two to four weeks for there to be any improvement, and many more before complete recovery, it is advisable to be patient and not to keep upping the dose during this time, especially since studies of elevation reveal that the same percentage of patients recover on 50 mg as on 200 mg, but many more on 200 mg are uncomfortable from side effects.

As mentioned earlier in describing the report of Drs. Brown and Harrison (see page 65), 79 percent of those who discontinued use of Prozac because of side effects were able to complete treatment with Zoloft. A switch to Prozac for those unable to tolerate Zoloft would also probably succeed, but since Prozac was released four years earlier than Zoloft, no one is doing research in the opposite direction. My colleagues and I have found that people who cannot tolerate one SSRI are often able to stand another. The minority who may feel "wired" on Prozac may feel less so on Zoloft. Prozac seems to make some people more anxious, restless, stimulated, and headachy than Zoloft. On the other hand, Zoloft may cause more hand tremors, drowsiness, diarrhea, and dry mouth. These differences are not very great, but may account for why someone could not tolerate one but could tolerate the other. When a person considers taking an SSRI, the issue of potential side effects should not guide him in his decision to take one of these agents over another. Your friend may say Prozac drove her up the wall, while Zoloft restored her health, but this report cannot help you, because your reaction may be the opposite.

Zoloft is effective in treating obsessive-compulsive disorder and all the other conditions I listed in the section on SSRIs in general, and on Prozac in particular. No SSRI has been found to be uniquely effective in treating a condition where the others are not.

Drug Interactions

Zoloft, like the other SSRIs, cannot be safely combined with an MAOI. In its favor, it has the reputation of posing the least risk of all the SSRIs for interactions with other drugs listed in the general section on SSRI interactions on pages 82 and 83. While this does not obviate the need for close supervision by your physician, it may allow you both to be a little less concerned.

Paxil

Paxil, the third SSRI to be released in the United States, is as effective as Prozac and Zoloft, or, put less delicately, is no more curative than the others. Its sales in 1995 were 45 percent above a year earlier and account for 21 percent of newer antidepressants sold in the United States. Claims that it acts faster remain unproven. Its marketing has focused on the speed and method by which it moves through the body after ingestion (so-called pharmacokinetics). What the physician in a hurry is supposed to believe is that Paxil, unlike the others, has no active metabolites, moves through the body fastest (pharmacokinetics), and is the most serotonin-selective. Thus, the doctor is able to adjust the patient's blood level of the drug more easily and to control it best. There are several problems with this scenario. First, blood levels of all SSRIs do not correlate with cure rate or side effect incidence, and therefore no clinician measures them. Second, Paxil may have no active metabolite, but Zoloft's so-called active metabolite is not very active. And finally, physicians think that due to the long duration of Prozac in the body, it is like stopping the *Titanic* if some bad side effect occurs, but there is no actual evidence that Prozac's side effects are more sinister or long-lasting than the other SSRIs. To counteract Paxil's no-active-metabolite purity, the makers of Zoloft have charged that it mucks up the liver enzymes that break down other drugs like desipramine, as well as Paxil itself, causing the blood levels of each to rise. Again, so what? The first problem is easily dealt with by giving lower desipramine doses, and the second makes no difference, since when the blood level of Paxil rises slowly over a week, nothing bad happens. The final point of the marketing is serotonin selectivity. It used to be that Zoloft's makers could say it was more serotonin-selective than Prozac, but now Paxil is the most serotonin-selective. Perhaps I am overly sensitive to advertising's attempts to influence me subconsciously, to make me feel more cultivated if I drink a certain beverage, more intelligent if I read a particular magazine, and more scientific a physician if I use the most specific of the selective serotonin reuptake inhibitors. In the back of my mind resonates nonspecific treatments that are nothing but placebos, that owe their effect to the enthusiasm and authority of the doctor rather than to the biological action of the drug itself. Doctors want, with laserlike accuracy, to kill the cancer cells and not the surrounding normal tissue, and psychiatrists want to manipulate the serotonin core of depression powerfully. Unfortunately, the serotonin levels are not the only factor to consider in comparing various drugs' efficacy. All the SSRIs are equally effective, and although on the ad scoreboard Paxil has beaten Prozac in serotonin selectivity 320 to 20, the all-around score, in fact, is tied.

Dosage

Most people can tolerate a starting dose of 20 mg of Paxil, which requires no change over the two to four weeks before the therapeutic effect begins to be felt, nor any for the whole duration on the drug. Some experience too many side effects initially and split the tablet in half or even into quarters until they get used to the side effects, and later are able to tolerate the full dosage. After a month on 20 mg, if the person has not recovered, the dose may be raised by 10 mg weekly until a daily maximum of 50 mg is reached.

Side Effects

In addition to causing the same side effects as the other SSRIs on the gastrointestinal tract, nervous system, and sexual functions, Paxil seems more likely to cause sweating, constipation, dry mouth, drowsiness, and fatigue, and less likely to cause nervousness and diarrhea. If, for example, nervousness has been a problem on Prozac, Paxil may be a sensible second choice.

The following is a story of someone who couldn't tolerate Prozac well, but was greatly helped by Paxil. John is forty-seven years old and has been very depressed since being fired from his job as an industrial engineer. He knows he should be mailing out résumés and networking with colleagues, but cannot get himself to do either. John has trouble falling and staying asleep, feels slowed down and without energy, and is convinced no one will hire him. He has black circles around his eyes; he barely speaks to his wife and snaps at his children. John cannot concentrate on anything he tries to read or write, and worries constantly about the future. After months of suffering, he took a friend's recommendation and came to see me. I started him on Prozac, and we began to talk about his illness and his life. After several weeks, he told me he could not stand the drug, that he was now up all night worrying and frightened, and that he felt tense and unable to relax. The anxiety of most depressed people is diminished by Prozac, but about 10 percent grow more upset from it, and become worse than before. John belonged to this minority.

I suggested he stop taking Prozac, wait a few days, and then begin half the normal 20-mg Paxil dose (the tablet is scored and easily divided). The reason for the lower dose is that Prozac would leave his system very slowly, and I did not want to wait until it was completely gone because of his suffering. Starting him on 10 mg of Paxil would be safe, and in a week I raised it to 20 mg. Two weeks later, he began to feel more energetic, to sleep better, and to make necessary phone calls. In a month, he was singing the praises of Paxil, as he actively pursued his job search.

The Properties of Paxil

Like Prozac and Zoloft, Paxil is safe and effective in the moderately to severely depressed, the anxious depressed, and the elderly. Since half of major depressives relapse in two years, and 80 to 90 percent who have suffered two episodes go on to have a third, prevention of further outbreaks of the illness is essential. Paxil, like the other SSRIs, decreases the relapse rate by about 30 percent.

Paxil is like Prozac in its blocking the liver enzyme metabolism of itself and other drugs, and like Zoloft in being shorter-acting. Its absorption is not affected by food or antacids. Except for the elderly and those with liver or kidney damage, who require lower amounts, most people start out on 20 mg in the morning and stay on it until recovery.

Paxil normalizes the sleep patterns in depressed people, unlike Prozac and Luvox, and helps those who take it in the morning to fall asleep at night and feel more rested the next day. In spite of this, the degree of insomnia as a side effect of all four SSRIs is about the same. Like Prozac, Paxil does not increase the drive toward suicide. In fact, they both lessen it.

If a patient has been on Paxil for months or more, suddenly discontinuing use of it is (of the SSRIs) most likely to cause very unpleasant withdrawal symptoms. These range from some odd and terrifying headaches and "brain shocks" to fatigue and/or insomnia. Flu-like symptoms of running nose, sweating, nausea, vomiting, diarrhea, and muscle pain may occur. Sometimes a migraine-like illness evolves, accompanied by severe dizziness and the seeing of small floating shapes. It is believed that Paxil is more likely to produce unpleasant withdrawal effects because of its shorter duration of action (it has a twenty-four-hour half-life) and lack of active metabolites. These are least likely to occur if the patient has taken Prozac, which is eliminated very slowly. Physical withdrawal symptoms have been reported to arise even when the dose of Paxil is tapered off very slowly over a week or two.

Drug Interactions

There are three levels of drug interactions with Paxil, as there are with Prozac and to a lesser extent with Zoloft: (1) the severe, (2) the moderate, and (3) the mild. The severe interactions involve the MAOIs Nardil and Parnate and any other drug that raises the level of serotonin, like tryptophan. The moderate interactions involve combinations with other drugs whose levels in the body are raised much higher than one might otherwise suspect. For example, if the normal dose of approximately 250 mg of desipramine were administered with Paxil or Prozac, it would be like giving 1,000 mg of the drug, which could cause serious toxicity. As mentioned earlier, an easy way around this problem is to give 50 mg of desipramine to people taking Paxil. This caution applies to other tricyclics and antipsychotics, like molindone.

The list of mild interactions is longest and constantly being added to. It includes those for all SSRIs, noted on pages 82 and 83, such as the increased danger of bleeding when on an anticoagulant, and the need for caution when taking antihistamines, anticonvulsants, antiarrhythmics, beta-blockers, and various psychiatric drugs. Remember to be careful when combining medications, and always consult your doctor before doing so.

Summary

Paxil is a safe and effective SSRI. It has the usual SSRI side effects on the gastrointestinal tract, the nervous system, and on sexual functioning. But it also shares the advantages of the SSRIs: (1) dosing is easy (one pill daily), (2) it is reasonably well tolerated, (3) it has no effect on the heart or blood pressure, (4) it has no effect on a person's ability to drive a car or other motor skills, and (5) there are few serious drug/drug interactions.

Luvox

In 1995, the Food and Drug Administration approved Luvox, which has been prescribed in Switzerland since 1983, five years before Prozac was released in the United States. The drug is used to treat depression in Europe, but is allowed in the United States only for obsessive-compulsive disorder (OCD); the matter of its possible use in treating depression here remains under further study. Nonetheless, any physician who wishes to prescribe it for depression can do so legally. In spite of the fact that Solvay, the European manufacturer of Luvox, asserts that 37,000 patients have been studied in controlled clinical trials and that by 1992, 4.5 million had been treated with the drug, there remains some doubt about the antidepressant efficacy of Luvox, because some of the small placebo-controlled studies found it positive and others negative. Thus, Solvay and Upjohn, the American manufacturer of Luvox, have the third approved medication for OCD following the tricyclic Anafranil, and the SSRI Prozac, but their application for its use as an antidepressant is still being reviewed by the FDA.

In addition to OCD, Luvox will undoubtedly be used to treat other repetitive behaviors (e.g., voyeurism, other sexual perversions and addictions, and behaviors exhibited by the autistic child). It will also be prescribed, as have other SSRIs, for Tourette's syndrome (characterized by tics, grunts, and obscenities), body dysmorphic disorders (feeling ugly or deformed although normal-looking), binge eating, self-injurious behavior, and pathologic jealousy.

Characteristics of Luvox

Its absorption is not affected by food, so half a dose of Luvox is eliminated by the body in fifteen hours, and it has no active metabolites (drug breakdown products). The dose range is 50 to 300 mg daily, and the manufacturer recommends that amounts above 100 mg be given in divided doses, with the larger one taken at bedtime. Presumably, this is because of the drug's rapid metabolism and perhaps also because nausea, which occurs in 40 percent of cases, will be lessened by not taking all the drug at once. The tablets are scored for easy division, and come in 50- and 100-mg sizes. The need to take it twice a day is a disadvantage of Luvox versus the other three SSRIs.

Side Effects

Luvox's side effects are typical of an SSRI: nausea, dyspepsia, abdominal pain, vomiting, sexual dysfunction, sleepiness, insomnia, nervousness, weakness, dizziness, constipation, and diarrhea. The drug usually does not cause weight gain, and is comparatively safe in overdose. Details of how its side effects compare with those of the other SSRIs have yet to be revealed. Like Paxil, with no active metabolites and a shorter half-life, it is more likely to cause a withdrawal syndrome if its use is suddenly discontinued.

Drug/Drug Interactions

Luvox interacts with tricyclic antidepressants, Coumadin (it raises the blood level of this anticoagulant, increasing the chance of bleeding), Tegretol, Dilantin, Inderal, methadone, and Valium (take Ativan instead). The drug does not seem to interact with the heart medicine digoxin, or with alcohol. Luvox cannot be given within two weeks of MAOIs like Nardil or Parnate. There can be danger to the heart in combining Luvox with the antihistamines Seldane and Hismanal and the antifungal agent Nizoral. This is a drug new to the United States, and its list of interactions, while not uniquely different from other SSRIs, is expanding rapidly. These are safe drugs, but their side effects and interactions must never be ignored.

Luvox and Other Drugs in
Obsessive-Compulsive Disorder (OCD)

As mentioned earlier, obsessions are unwanted, usually horrific thoughts, impulses, and images that are experienced by the sufferer as products of his own mind which are inappropriate and should be suppressed, and that cause anxiety. Behavioral and mental compulsions include hand-washing, arranging and checking (e.g., is the gas off?) behaviors, and mental acts (e.g., counting, endlessly reviewing conversations for hidden meaning), useless repetitions that a person is driven to perform to decrease stress or magically prevent a dreaded event. These obsessions and compulsions cause marked distress, are time-consuming (more than an hour a day), or interfere with social or occupational functioning.

The word *compulsive* is used in everyday parlance to refer to excessive eating, drinking, sex, and gambling, but these activities are experienced as pleasurable, whereas true compulsions are not. Unlike the obsessive-compulsive personality (OCP), who is proud of his orderliness, punctuality, and frugality, the OCD experiences his thoughts and impulses as disgusting, horrific, and to be controlled.

On April 25, 1994, Michael Miller, writing in the *Wall Street Journal*, warned of an advertising plot by "two giant companies, Upjohn and Solvay," makers of Luvox, to reach the large numbers of OCD sufferers who go undiagnosed and untreated in order to increase sale of this drug. The author speaks of the packaging and marketing of diseases to people, pointing out that the Food and Drug Administration prohibits drug advertising aimed directly at patients. These two companies spent $1 million, Miller reported, to hire a public relations firm to promote a slogan about "unlocking the Captive Mind" to doctors, patients, and their families. They also funded Dr. Robert DuPont, Mr. Miller continues, to study the annual economic costs of OCD, and the preliminary conclusion was between $8 and $10 billion. Next, Miller noted that another psychiatrist, Wayne Goodman of the University of Florida, was preparing a short quiz for consumers to determine if they have signs of OCD. A strategy like this will most likely work, if the experience with attention deficit hyperactivity disorder (ADHD) is any guide. I answered a questionnaire in *The New York Times Book Review* advertising a popular book on the subject, and found I had seventeen positive signs for the disorder out of twenty. It is no accident that sales of Ritalin, used to treat this condition, have sharply increased in the past year. I do not mean to imply that ADHD is not real, any more than OCD is not one of the most painful illnesses imaginable. I am referring instead to the practice of marketing the mildest forms of these conditions to the public. Upjohn and Solvay are now looking for a celebrity sufferer of OCD to advertise it. Perhaps their difficulty in finding one means that the true disorder is rare after all, and that if a person really had it, he would be socially isolated, celibate, and spending days in meaningless activities, rather than famous.

All the SSRIs are effective in treating OCD, two are officially recognized by the Food and Drug Administration (Prozac and Luvox), and only one is solely for OCD (Luvox). Does this make Luvox the best choice? There is no evidence that Luvox is more effective in treating OCD than other SSRIs. If you nonetheless decide to try it, give it three months to work. About one third to half of those taking it improve. Those who get better need to keep taking the drug or they will relapse, and they tend not to get completely well. For those who do not completely recover, the best therapy (in addition to the drug) is behavioral therapy, which directly exposes them to the terrifying dirt or germ, prevents them from washing, and teaches them to control their anxiety and calm themselves. Confronting pictures of or imagining the terrifying situation does not work as well as real contact.

If a person with OCD decides to try Paxil, 40 to 60 mg works better than the usual 20-mg dose. For Zoloft, a maximum dose of 200 mg may be necessary. Higher doses of Prozac (40 to 80 mg) also seem to be more effective than the standard 20 mg. Occasionally, a person will do better on a lower than usual SSRI dosage. If an OCD sufferer also has tics (blinking, shoulder-shrugging, throat-clearing), a low dose of an antipsychotic drug like Haldol added to Luvox can be helpful.

Summary

Luvox is a new old drug, new (1995) to America, but old (1983) to Europe. The twelve-year-plus experience with it abroad makes me feel safer with it than I normally would with a brand-new medication. Its drawbacks are that it must be used twice daily (instead of once) because of its being rapidly metabolized, and that there is some question about its effectiveness in treating depression. Because it is marketed specifically for OCD, I would applaud a more powerful action in obsessive-compulsive disorder than that of the tricyclic Anafranil or the other three SSRIs, but so far there is no evidence of this. As a psychiatrist, I do not plan to prescribe it until its superiority for OCD is established.

Are There Any Differences in Side Effects Among the SSRIs?

In large studies, statistically significant differences among the SSRIs are difficult to show, and the drugs seem very much alike. Paxil causes the least diarrhea and most constipation among the three, and therefore, if a person cannot tolerate the loose stools caused by Prozac or Zoloft, Paxil is a reasonable alternative. If the dry mouth caused by Zoloft or Paxil is a problem, perhaps a change to Prozac would help. Zoloft and Paxil probably cause less nervousness than Prozac, but Paxil may cause more fatigue and drowsiness. If you are wired from Prozac, try Paxil; if you are sluggish from Paxil, try Prozac.

I have constructed a table comparing the side effects of the three drugs based on averages from a number of studies. Most of the adverse reactions occur less than 10 percent of the time, and many of them are minor and disappear in a few weeks. The table is based on a system of one to four plus signs, with one being the least likelihood of a side effect, and four being the most.

Possible Side Effect Differences Among the SSRIs

	Prozac	Zoloft	Paxil
Nervousness	++++	+++	+++
Drowsiness and fatigue	+	+	++
Dry mouth and constipation	+	++	+++
Weight gain	+	+	+
Diarrhea	++	+++	+
Sweating	++	++	+++

It has been my experience that Prozac and Paxil are the most dissimilar in terms of the side effects they produce, and Zoloft has the fewest interactions with other drugs.

SSRI Summary

There are three reasons why the SSRIs as a class are now the most widely prescribed antidepressants: the ease of taking them, their tolerability, and their safety in overdose.

Dosage

The one-pill-a-day starting dose is usually also the maximum dose. Gone is the need, in most instances, to gradually elevate drug intake from one to twelve tablets a day, as with the tricyclic antidepressants. Three of the four new antidepressants described in the next chapter (Wellbutrin, Effexor, Serzone, not Remeron) must be taken more than once a day.

Tolerability

Although 20 percent of people who start on an SSRI stop taking it within weeks, and another 15 percent within months, because of side effects, the large majority suffer little or no discomfort from them. These drugs do not interfere with driving and other skilled tasks, and do not increase the effects of alcohol. Thus, more people complete the treatment at full dosage for an acute depressive episode, and those who need to are able to continue long-term therapy to prevent relapse. The gastrointestinal side effects, at first troubling to some, usually can be tolerated and eventually subside, as do the side effects on the central nervous system, such as anxiety and sleep disturbance. Unfortunately, the sexual difficulties induced by the SSRIs are fairly common, occurring in 30 to 50 or more percent by some estimates, and for many physicians and patients constitute the prime weakness of these agents. The list of rare side effects and drug/drug interactions is growing, as more experience with these medications is gathered, making it essential that you keep in touch with your prescribing physician.

Safety in Overdose

The illness of depression is often accompanied by suicidal thoughts and impulses, as well as actual suicide attempts. The SSRIs are fairly safe in overdose, which allows the doctor to prescribe adequate amounts without excessive fear. The danger of suicide with tricyclic antidepressants is one of the reasons they were given in too small doses, and thus did not produce a full therapeutic effect.

SSRIs, in spite of an early erroneous report, do not increase suicidal ideas, impulses, and actions. In overdose, they do not affect the heart, pulse rate, or blood pressure, nor do they cause any severe nervous system response (e.g., seizure, coma), and as a result, very few deaths from SSRI overdose occur.

If Prozac, Zoloft, Paxil, and Luvox are so good, why are there three more chapters in this book describing even more antidepressants? The answer has to do with efficacy and side effects. About 30 percent of the people who try them do not respond to SSRIs, and perhaps another 20 percent are improved, but not completely cured. Furthermore, the rate of response and cure is too slow, so that the search for faster relief must continue. And finally, the SSRIs are not tolerated by everyone (perhaps 35 percent), the main reason being the sexual side effects.

CHAPTER 4

The New Antidepressants: Wellbutrin, Effexor, Serzone, and Remeron

There are four other new antidepressants that are currently available: Wellbutrin, Effexor, Serzone, and Remeron. New drugs are like new cars; they look good, but no one knows how they will wear. Wellbutrin was subject to a recall by its manufacturer weeks after its initial release in 1986, and its image has still not completely recovered. Effexor has not become a popular model because it requires too much maintenance. Not only must it be taken more than once a day, but the patient's blood pressure must be regularly monitored in order to detect the hypertension the drug sometimes causes. Serzone still looks good, but may, though it has an advantage over the SSRIs in not causing insomnia and anxiety, make too many people dizzy, light-headed, drowsy, and fatigued. Or it may not. There is always curiosity about (and fear of) the new. Remeron, the newest of all, also may make too many feel drugged and fatigued, and also may cause weight gain and threaten the white blood cell count.

The ongoing appetite for new antidepressants exists because of the failures of the old ones. While the majority of people taking them have been helped, 30 percent do not respond, and an additional 20 percent are not completely cured. Also, the episodic nature of depression allows the sufferer to take a new drug after a new occurrence. Side effects cause 20 percent to go off the first antidepressant soon after starting, and an additional 15 percent to discontinue it within a year. It is estimated that if you are depressed, your first medication will fail you about 40 percent of the time, either because it does not work or because it makes you too uncomfortable. This leaves the market wide open for agents that are presumably more effective or better tolerated. It is good to have Wellbutrin, Effexor, Serzone, and Remeron as alternatives for those who have not been helped by or cannot tolerate the SSRIs.

Wellbutrin

Wellbutrin was about to be released in 1986, two years before Prozac, as an effective antidepressant with the same advantages over tricyclics as the SSRIs—namely, less dry mouth, blurred vision, constipation, weight gain, drop in blood pressure, or danger to the heart. In a 1986 prerelease study, the drug caused four grand mal seizures in 55 nondepressed bulimic women, and it was withdrawn for further testing. Burroughs Wellcome, the manufacturer of Wellbutrin, went on to study the frequency of Wellbutrin-induced seizures in 3,000 depressed patients, and found that if it was given in a maximum amount of 150 mg three times a day up to 450 mg total daily, the seizure rate was roughly comparable to that with other antidepressants. The reason for the 150-mg ceiling for a given dose is that seizures are significantly dose-related, and most likely to occur after a given dose or dose change. Missed doses should not be "doubled up" next time the drug is taken. At 1 in 250, the seizure rate was about the same as with the tricyclics. The seizure rate for all patients on Prozac in a similar premarketing study was 1 in 500, which is not very different, while that for Zoloft and Paxil was less than 1 in 1,000. Seizures in tricyclics occur in 1 out of 200 patients taking average doses of 150 mg a day. The incidence of seizures in a survey of patients not on antidepressants in general practice in Britain was 0.4 percent, or the same 1 in 250 as that found for Wellbutrin. It has been concluded that seizures are unlikely to occur if Wellbutrin is given in divided doses of less than 150 mg at a time to people who are *not* bulimic and do not possess other predisposing factors for seizures, such as a history of epilepsy, alcoholism, head trauma, brain tumor, fever, or drugs lowering the seizure threshold (e.g., tricyclics, antipsychotics, lithium, short-acting benzodiazepines like Halcion and Xanax). The drug was rereleased three years later, in 1989. But the seizure history limited its use until only recently, when it was found that those who take it are unlikely to experience drug-related impairment of their sexual functioning. Maybe it was more acceptable than the SSRIs after all. Nonetheless, the need to raise the dose slowly and to take as many as nine pills daily in three divided doses makes it cumbersome to use. To overcome this handicap, the manufacturer is researching a sustained release form of the drug that can be taken only once a day. The necessity of gradually elevating the dose would remain, but would be simpler on a once-daily basis.

How Wellbutrin actually works is unknown. This makes it different from all other antidepressants in use, and makes it desirable, perhaps, for people who are not helped by other drugs.

The Effectiveness of Wellbutrin

Wellbutrin is no more curative than other new antidepressants, but it has been better studied. Although it is an activating drug like Prozac, it also reduces anxiety, even in those depressed patients who are anxious before treatment. It can be safely taken by people with heart disease, high blood pressure, and other illnesses. In depressives who neither respond to nor can tolerate other drugs, Wellbutrin has been effective in from a half to two thirds of cases. It has been found effective in people who don't respond to the tricyclics. Patients who have suffered sexual side effects on SSRIs often do well on Wellbutrin. Sporadic studies, in need of controlled confirmation, suggest that Wellbutrin does not destabilize the moods of bipolar depressives, as do other antidepressants, tipping fewer into mania or rapid cycling (more than four manic or depressive episodes per year). The drug has also been used (but is not FDA-approved) to effectively treat chronic fatigue syndrome. It is said *not* to be effective in treating depression associated with panic disorder, in pure panic disorder, or in obsessive-compulsive disorder.

One bright example of a case in which Wellbutrin worked where eight other antidepressants had failed is a forty-four-year-old patient of mine. Bob had suffered six-month-long major depressive episodes every two years since his late teens. Although he had never been hospitalized, they succeeded in destroying his life, interrupting his education so that it took ten years for him to complete his course in accounting, and ruined all his jobs. Although he finally completed his course work, he had not been able to pass his certified public accounting (CPA) test and was working part-time as a bartender. The ten major depressive episodes that came over him without apparent cause had resulted in his losing track of most of his friends, and all but a few family members. When he was ill, he had no appetite, could not sleep, would burst into tears without cause, was unable to concentrate on what he read, and had no energy to work. The fact that at those times his sex drive was zero seemed minor. He had been treated without much success with five tricyclic antidepressants (Elavil, Tofranil, desipramine, Pamelor, and Sinequan) as well as three different SSRIs (Prozac, Zoloft, and Paxil). Not only had they failed him in the acute phase, they had not been able to prevent his biannual recurrences. Wellbutrin not only sped recovery from his eleventh episode, it prevented relapse for four years. Although it is too early to pronounce him cured forever, the drug has spared him long enough so far that he has been able to get a better job, save money, get married, and buy a home. For Bob, Wellbutrin has worked a minor miracle.

Dosage

One hundred milligrams of Wellbutrin is taken in the morning and evening for the first three days, and on the fourth, a midday 100-mg tablet is added. If a dose is forgotten, it cannot be corrected by doubling the next amount because of the danger of seizure induction. The maximum dosage for those not responsive to less is 150 mg three times a day, although 300 mg is usually enough.

Side Effects

When it was originally released in 1986, two years before Prozac, Wellbutrin was set to be the best antidepressant because it produced the fewest side effects. It had the tricyclics beat because it caused less or no sedation, postural hypotension, dry mouth, sweating, blurred vision, constipation, weight gain, sexual dysfunction, rapid pulse, urinary retention, enhancement of alcohol or other central nervous system depressants, and disturbances of memory. But because the release of Wellbutrin was delayed for three years due to its seizure problem, it was not available in 1988 when Prozac was released, offering *almost* the same list of benefits. Prozac quickly became number one in the nation and the world. Wellbutrin is now, as I noted earlier, making a modest comeback against Prozac because of its much lower incidence of sexual side effects. Neither Wellbutrin nor the SSRIs adversely affect the heart, and both are safe in overdose.

The most common side effects of Wellbutrin are gastrointestinal and stimulatory, just as with Prozac. Patients may suffer nausea and mild dry mouth, but those who cannot tolerate Wellbutrin usually cannot because of its stimulatory effects, which they find unbearable. Agitation, insomnia, anxiety, and tremors are the reasons for the rare premature discontinuation of treatment. Most often the stimulatory effects occur early in treatment, soon gradually subside, and are less of a problem if the dose is low at first and very slowly raised. Because of its stimulatory effects, Wellbutrin should not be taken at bedtime. Sleep disturbance due to depression responds slowly to Wellbutrin, because all antidepressants take weeks to act, and a sleeping pill may be necessary at the beginning of treatment. In 5 to 10 percent of the women who take it, Wellbutrin can disrupt menstruation.

Wellbutrin's Lower Incidence of Sexual Dysfunction

Estimates of sexual dysfunction on Prozac range from 2 to 75 percent. In a study of thirty-one patients who had had difficulty with orgasm on Prozac and who were taken off all psychiatric medications for two weeks and then put on Wellbutrin for at least four weeks, 84 percent reported improved orgasm, more sexual satisfaction, and increased desire. Wellbutrin never worsened orgasmic function. Its most common side effects were anxiety, agitation, nausea, constipation, and headaches. Because this study was not blinded (both the patients and the doctors knew the treatment being given), the patients' expectations may have influenced the outcome. Nonetheless, it seems to support the notion that Wellbutrin does not interfere with sexual functioning. Another pair of researchers (E. A. Gardner and J. A. Johnston) found that diminished sexual desire resulting from antidepressants went away when Wellbutrin was substituted. Diminished sexual desire is often caused by depression as well as the drug treating it, whereas inhibition or absence of ejaculation or of orgasm is due not to the illness but to the antidepressant drug. While Wellbutrin improves or does not harm all of these sexual functions, its effect on desire is harder to determine.

Overdose

Overdose deaths from Wellbutrin are extremely rare. About one third of those who overdose develop seizures but recover.

Side Effects Compared to the SSRIs

The side effect frequency with Wellbutrin is low, and there are few significant differences between Wellbutrin and the SSRIs. Wellbutrin causes more nervousness and palpitations, and less fatigue, while the SSRIs cause more nausea and diarrhea. Wellbutrin causes more dry mouth and constipation, but these are usually mild. Weakness is more common with the SSRIs. The side effect differences between the drugs have not yet been carefully compared in a double-blind study.

Drug/Drug Interactions

In general, Wellbutrin's drug/drug interactions are minimal. MAOIs (Nardil, Parnate) are absolutely not to be taken with Wellbutrin. Its combination with the Parkinson's disease drug levodopa should be cautious, because of stimulatory and gastrointestinal side effects. Wellbutrin should be used with great caution or not at all with drugs that lower the seizure threshold (e.g., other antidepressants, alcohol, short-acting benzodiazepines such as Xanax). Because of Wellbutrin's narrow dose range (below 225 mg, it has no effect, and above 450 mg, there is a danger of convulsions), other drugs that raise or lower its blood level can be dangerous. Thus, if you have been taking Prozac and want to switch, remember that Prozac leaves the body slowly and raises the level of Wellbutrin. Thus, you should wait two weeks before starting to take Wellbutrin. It is safe to give Wellbutrin with clonidine, antiarrhythmic drugs, Coumadin, and digitalis.

Summary

In 1994, Prozac's sales were $1.3 billion, and Wellbutrin's (after a 30 percent growth because of its low sexual side effects) $75 million. The reasons for this fifteen-fold discrepancy lie not in the drugs' effectiveness or side effect patterns, which are the same, but in fear of Wellbutrin-induced seizures and the need to take the drug three times a day. When Wellbutrin is taken at the clinically effective dose of no more than 450 mg a day, its seizure rate is 4 in 1,000, quite similar to the 2 in 1,000 of Prozac, and the 3 in 1,000 of Paxil. The sustained-release form is expected to be available soon, and will allow Wellbutrin to be taken once daily, and perhaps reduce the danger of seizures by lowering peak plasma levels. Wellbutrin is a safe and effective antidepressant, giving people the choice between the convenient, once-daily dosage offered by the SSRIs, accompanied by a high incidence of sexual dysfunction, and an inconvenient, three-times-daily dosage with few sexual side effects.

Effexor

In 1994, Effexor was introduced by Wyeth-Ayerst as "Prozac with a punch," because of its action not only as an SSRI but also as a norepinephrine reuptake inhibitor (NERI), giving it a double-barreled impact on depression. The manufacturer presented it as having few side effects, like the SSRIs, accompanied by greater efficacy.

Effexor's Effectiveness

Some studies have shown that Effexor is faster-acting and more effective than Prozac and the other new antidepressants, but there is much skepticism about these claims. Over the last forty years, several antidepressant drugs have initially promised quicker relief, only to later fail to provide it. The search for relief in a matter of days rather than weeks or months is fueled by not only the suffering of patients and their families from this painful illness, but also the suicide rate of 15 percent among depressives. In prerelease studies of Effexor, the rate at which the dose was raised was faster than would be likely in normal clinical practice. This causes a faster response to the drug, but also more side effects.

Effexor is said to be more effective than other new antidepressants in hospitalized depressives. In one recent study, it was found to be better than Prozac in the treatment of severely depressed inpatients. This is a new drug, and more studies are necessary before it can be said with confidence that Effexor is truly more powerful in this group of patients. This power, if it exists, may be due to the physician's willingness to push doses higher and monitor blood pressure readings more closely in the hospital than is practical with people outside it. Thus, while Effexor's superiority to the SSRIs is an interesting point (if true), it may have little relevance for the average depressed outpatient. But if a person is suffering from a severe, otherwise unresponsive depression, then careful dose elevation to 375 mg per day, coupled with a willingness to carefully watch blood pressure and tolerate possible nausea, anxiety, insomnia, and sexual side effects, may yield the relief not available from other antidepressants.

It is believed that Effexor initially acts primarily as an SSRI, and that its norepinephrine effect occurs at higher doses. This explains the responsiveness at higher amounts of those not helped at lesser ones.

The Effexor believers regard the drug as faster-acting, more effective in the severely ill inpatient, and able to help a third or more of those refractory to other drugs and treatment. While there are scraps of evidence to back all this up, they are extremely meager. The skeptics are quick to point out marketing tricks, such as comparing a new drug like Effexor with the old tricyclics at inadequate doses, so that the new agent will appear more effective, and the practice of comparing it to tricyclics with more side effects (e.g., Elavil and Tofranil) rather than to those with fewer (e.g., desipramine, Pamelor), so that the new agent will appear less toxic. Remember: for a drug to be released, all it need do is be more effective than a placebo and neither kill anyone nor cause other unacceptable toxicity. Comparing it in detail with existing drugs in its class comes much later, if ever. I hope Effexor is better, as its advocates claim. There clearly is a need for it.

Dosage

Effexor is started at 37.5 mg once or twice a day and taken with food, then moved up every four days until a total of 150 mg is reached. When necessary, the amount can be gradually raised further every four days to 225 mg per day, taken in two or three divided doses. For severely depressed patients, 350 mg daily is sometimes prescribed.

Hypertension

As Wellbutrin's reputation has been tainted by the risk of seizures, so has Effexor's been by a connection with hypertension. In both cases, the hype is worse than the reality, but it is enough to dampen enthusiasm about each. Effexor has been shown to raise blood pressure primarily at doses over 225 mg a day. The increase is small and dose-related. For example, if your blood pressure were 120/80 and you were taking 375 mg per day of Effexor, your blood pressure would increase by only 8 points.

In clinical trials, patients who are not medically healthy are typically excluded, and so the effect of Effexor on people with high blood pressure was not studied. Once hypertension occurs, the patient can be treated with an antihypertension drug, have the Effexor dose reduced, or change to another antidepressant. Hypertension, when it occurs, does so within two months of a given dose of Effexor having been established, and it is during this two-month period that patients require closest observation. People taking more than 225 mg a day of Effexor must take their blood pressure or have it taken, regularly. With seven other new antidepressants and more than a dozen old ones, it is easy to see why Effexor is often not the first to be used.

Other Adverse Effects

Effexor is safe, even in overdose, from which people have survived thousands of milligrams without serious consequences. In fact, the nausea and vomiting that is induced by overdose serves to decrease the severity of the consequences.

The nausea, nervousness, dizziness, and sleepiness caused by Effexor at its starting dose of 37.5 or 75 mg a day is quite similar to the side effects of SSRIs. The incidence of side effects increases as the dose is raised. At the maximum dosage of 375 mg a day, about 40 percent of people taking the drug are nauseous, 13 percent sweating, 20 percent sleepy, 20 percent dizzy, and 10 percent suffer tremors. At lower doses, these unpleasant reactions are much less common. The abnormal ejaculation/orgasm, impotence, and lowered sexual desire caused by Effexor are the same as that for the SSRIs.

Drug Interactions

Just as with the SSRIs, Effexor should not be taken with an MAOI. It should not be started for fourteen days after use of an MAOI is stopped, but, because of its short stay in the body, an MAOI can be taken seven days after use of Effexor is discontinued. Effexor does not seem to raise the blood levels of psychoactive drugs like the tricyclic desipramine, antipsychotics, and Tegretol. Tagamet taken together with Effexor raises Effexor's blood levels, which may mean that lower doses of Effexor will have to be used. No known interaction occurs between Effexor and lithium, alcohol, or benzodiazepines.

When drugs are as new as Effexor is, their interactions are

primarily theoretical and predicted by the test tube. Only with experience do the clinically relevant interactions become apparent. Until we know more, caution should be used when combining Effexor with other drugs, and as with all medications, be sure to consult your physician before doing so.

Summary

Effexor seems a safe and effective antidepressant. The assertion that it is better than Prozac, because it affects two neurotransmitters (serotonin and norepinephrine), rather than one, remains unproven. Claims that it acts in a matter of days instead of weeks to combat depression may be an artifact of pushing high doses in time-limited trials with too little regard for the greater number of side effects thus caused. Proof for the notion that it is more effective in severely depressed patients also requires more than a study or two. And finally, the uncontrolled trial indicating that one third of previously untreatable depressives were helped by Effexor needs placebo-controlled replications, because new drugs usually help people due to the enthusiasm of both doctors and patients. If Effexor is truly more effective, especially in those who have not previously been helped by other treatments, then the fact that it must be taken more than once a day, that its dose must be slowly raised, and that blood pressure must be carefully monitored, is a small price to pay for relief from pain and suffering caused by depression.

Serzone

Serzone, released in 1995, is one of the newest antidepressants. It is similar in structure to Desyrel, a drug that has many negative side effects, including drowsiness and faintness.

Serzone, like the SSRIs, prevents serotonin reuptake, but it has a broader action, as does Effexor, in that it also blocks the reuptake of norepinephrine. Unlike the other new anti-depressants, it has a third action, its most powerful, also on the serotonin synapse: it blocks one of the targets of serotonin, and perhaps that is why it does not make people sleepless, anxious, and sexless, as the SSRIs do. It is a little hard to understand how a drug that simultaneously elevates the level of serotonin and blocks its target works, but I have begun to regard the serotonin synapse the same way I think of my radio when it does not work—I hit it and it often starts broadcasting again. I have begun to believe that is what these antidepressants do to the synapse—they hit it.

Serzone's Effectiveness

Serzone's effectiveness is equal to that of the tricyclic Tofranil and the SSRIs. The higher the dose of Serzone taken, the stronger its antidepressant power—up to 500 mg a day. At 600 mg a day, however, its effectiveness is weakened to that of a placebo. Since only nonresponders (those who don't get better on the drug) got the 600-mg dose in the studies, this finding may have little meaning beyond the fact that those who do not improve on 500 mg probably will not do so on 600 mg either, and so there is no advantage in raising the dose above 500 mg.

Within one week of starting Serzone, patients will notice an improvement in sleep and anxiety symptoms. The complete antidepressant response is no faster than that with other drugs. The value of Serzone in severe hospitalized patients requires further research. Continued treatment with Serzone produces protection against relapse comparable to that with other antidepressants.

Dosage

Serzone is started at 100 mg twice a day, and one week later is increased to 300 mg a day, which is taken as 150 mg twice or 100 mg three times. This is usually enough, but the dose can gradually be raised to a maximum of 500 mg a day. A greater response is expected at higher doses for those who do not improve initially.

Side Effects

Serzone, like the other modern antidepressants, has no ill effect on the heart, even in overdosage. Dizziness, drowsiness, weakness, and lack of energy are its most common side effects, and occur more often than with any of the other new drugs, except perhaps Remeron. In one study A. Feiger et al. found Serzone to cause dizziness in 32 percent versus 7 percent on Zoloft. The reason for this is believed to be that it is the only one of the new drugs that blocks one of the serotonin receptors (serotonin-2) as well as the serotonin uptake pump. People are given the choice of being dizzy and sleepy or sexless, depending on whether they take Serzone or an SSRI.

Fortunately, the modifications to its parent, Desyrel, have eliminated much of the drowsy, drugged feeling caused by the older compound. Desyrel also caused priapism (a permanent erection) in one of six thousand males treated. Although this has not yet been reported with Serzone, it may still happen.

The clear advantage of Serzone over the SSRIs, Wellbutrin, and Effexor is that it causes less sweating, anxiety, sleeplessness, and diarrhea. In fact, not only does the drug excel in these respects, it is better than a placebo, which means that it effectively combats anxiety in those who are depressed. Since a large number of depressed people are also anxious, this offers a distinct advantage. Also, since many require the help of a sleeping pill for several weeks until the nonsedating SSRI, Wellbutrin, or Effexor exerts its antidepressant action, Serzone's action as a sleep aid may be another advantage.

Serzone and Sex

So far, it looks like Serzone has a lower incidence of sexual side effects than the other antidepressants. One reason to withhold complete confidence in this assertion is that most studies are conducted for six weeks, and sexual side effects may occur after that initial six-week period. In addition, those who are seriously depressed do not care about sex or anything else, and may not report sexual dysfunction until they have recovered and become interested in sex again, and then find they cannot perform. There is also a difference between the ways in which men and women report sexual side effects. When a drug interferes with their sexual functioning, men are likely to report this side effect without being asked. Males complain spontaneously when they cannot get an erection or have difficulty ejaculating. Women, on the other hand, often attribute their loss of sexual interest or performance not to the drug but rather to being overworked or irritated with their husband or lover. Thus, they tend not to spontaneously report sexual side effects, and if the researchers do not specifically ask, they will underreport these side effects.

Wellbutrin is a drug to which you can change if the SSRIs have harmed your sexual functioning. Desyrel, the parent of Serzone, was found not to harm, and perhaps even to encourage, the sexual drive of women. In some cases, it went too far with men, producing permanent erection (priapism). So far it seems that Serzone is fulfilling its early promise as an effective antidepressant which does not harm sexual functioning.

Serzone/Drug Interactions

The warning not to combine certain drugs with MAOIs extends to Serzone, although there is less potential danger than with the other antidepressants. Caution should be used when combining this drug with the antihistamines Seldane and Hismanal because of the unlikely but possible danger of increasing their blood levels, thus interfering with heart rhythm, which potentially can lead to ventricular tachycardia and death. The combination of these drugs with the anti-fungal agent Nizoral or others and with the gastrointestinal agent Propulsid (cisapride) could also be toxic to the heart. The levels of Xanax and Halcion are raised four times by combining these drugs with Serzone. Serzone does not affect the asthma drug theophylline (Asbron) or the anticoagulant warfarin (Coumadin) or the anticonvulsant phenytoin (Dilantin). It does not increase the effects of alcohol and sedatives.

Summary

At the time of this writing, Serzone has been on the market for less than two years. For a drug to be made available, it only has to be effective in six-week studies and not obviously dangerous. To get to really know a drug takes a long time, and even after over thirty years, some potentially serious effects of Tofranil and Elavil on the heart remain inadequately investigated. Those whose previous antidepressant drug experience has been negative may be moved by their pain to try this new medication. For those who have been successfully helped in the past by another drug without too many side effects, it is probably sensible to take the same one again.

If the initial promise of Serzone as a drug that will not cause agitation, insomnia, or sexual dysfunction holds up, and if it does not make too many feel weak and dizzy, there will be an important role for this drug.

Remeron

Remeron, released in 1996, is a brand-new antidepressant, unrelated to the SSRIs or other antidepressants. Because of its newness it is the only drug of this type with which I do not have extensive firsthand clinical experience.

Remeron enhances the amount of both serotonin and nor-epinephrine released into the synapse, but also blocks some of the target receptors of serotonin, which may account for why it, like Serzone, does not cause as much insomnia, anxiety, and sexual disturbance as the SSRIs. In addition, it affects several other neurotransmitters, which cause weight gain and mild sleepiness.

Remeron's Effectiveness

Five studies have shown Remeron's effectiveness in depressed patients equal to that of the tricyclic Elavil and superior to placebo, in the standard six-week controlled trials required by the Food and Drug Administration. As with the other new antidepressants, especially at the time of FDA approval, the main evidence of effectiveness has been obtained in outpatients. The smaller number of inpatient (and most likely, more seriously ill) depressives studied shows Remeron equal to other antidepressants, but more research is necessary.

Dosage

The recommended starting dose is one 15-mg tablet at bedtime, which if ineffective after two to four weeks can be raised gradually to 45 mg or more. Dosages recommended on release of a new drug are frequently modified as clinical experience with it grows. Thus, the starting 15 mg may in time be raised or lowered. The relationship between dosage and antidepressant response has not yet been established. Nonetheless, Remeron has the advantage of once-a-day dosage like the SSRIs and unlike Wellbutrin, Effexor, and Serzone. The drug is available in 15- and 30-mg scored tablets.

Side Effects

Remeron makes more than half of those who take it sleepy, especially in the first week of treatment, thus the recommendation that it be taken at bedtime. Going to work the next morning or being alert will probably not be a problem because its sedative effect is not very strong. Nonetheless, care should be taken when driving. Sleepiness from antidepressants relieves insomnia at night and is usually gone the next day, especially after several weeks. Remeron causes about 10 percent to feel weakness and lack of energy. Appetite increase was reported in 17 percent and weight gain in 12 percent of patients in the brief six-week controlled studies, but may be more of a problem during the months and years of normal clinical usage. Dry mouth is a common (25 percent) early side effect of Remeron, but it is usually mild and subsides in a few weeks.

Remeron and Sex

In the premarketing assessment of 2,796 patients, abnormal ejaculation was found to be rare (fewer than 1/1,000 patients), impotence infrequent (1/100 to 1/1,000 patients) and no mention is made of loss of sexual drive or orgasm potential. While it is likely that the sexual side effects will be less than those caused by the SSRIs, it is almost certain there will be more than reported in the six-week prerelease studies.

Other Adverse Effects

Severe Decrease in White Blood Cell Count

Three patients (1.1 per thousand) developed white counts below 500 (normal 3,800) during prerelease clinical trials. This occurrence is rare, but if you get a sore throat, fever, or other sign of infection, your doctor should test your blood. If the count is low, Remeron must be discontinued. While most antidepressant drugs lower the white count on rare occasions, none warn of its most severe form, agranulocytosis (a count below 500), in bold type in the PDR. The manufacturer does not advise periodic, routine blood counts, but suggests doing one should a fever or sign of infection occur. The need to go for a blood count with every winter sore throat and fever can be easily forgotten by doctor and patient. Since Remeron offers no clear advantage over the other new antidepressants, I do not plan to use it as a first-line drug until more is known about its white blood count dangers. I would use it with extreme care only after all other treatments had failed.

MAO Inhibitors

As with all the other new antidepressants, the manufacturer recommends Remeron not be used in combination with an MAOI.

Cholesterol Increases

Fifteen percent of patients treated with Remeron had up to a 20 percent increase of their nonfasting cholesterol level. I do not know how much of a problem this will prove to be, but it is something to be alert about when taking the drug for a long time.

Discontinuation of Treatment

Patients having to discontinue treatment within six weeks because of adverse effects number the same 16 percent occurring with other new antidepressants, and no doubt the number would have risen if observations had continued for a whole year, perhaps to the 30 to 35 percent level seen with other of these drugs. Remeron causes sleepiness, weight gain, dizziness, dry mouth, constipation, feelings of weakness, and debility, which lead to discontinuation in six weeks, and perhaps unknown late-occurring side effects, which would cause more patients to stop.

Drug Interactions

Remeron, because of its sedative side effects, probably will not mix very well with alcohol or Valium. Like all new antidepressants, it should not be taken with MAO inhibitors. Its effect on the liver and resulting interaction with other drugs is still theoretical and said by the manufacturer to be minimal, but all should be alert to the possibility as experience with Remeron grows.

Overdose

Experience with Remeron is sparse in this area. Overdose causes drowsiness, memory impairment, disorientation, rapid pulse, but so far there are no reports of serious effects on the heart or brain.

Summary

The search for more effective and better tolerated antidepressants goes on. The SSRIs cause gastrointestinal upset, agitation, insomnia, and interfere with sexual functioning. So far none of their successors has been more effective, and all have side effects, only different ones. Remeron is the first (perhaps the last) member of a new class of drugs, the noradrenaline (norepinephrine) and serotonin specific (*not* reuptake inhibitor) antidepressants (NaSSAs). It is no more effective than the SSRIs, probably causes fewer sexual side effects, but substitutes the danger of weight gain, mild dry mouth, drowsiness, dizziness, and weakness (hopefully mild and transitory), and worry about the rare danger of white blood cell destruction, resulting in potentially life-threatening infections.

The following conclusions can be drawn about these new drugs:

- They are all equally effective.
- More work will be required to prove the claim that Effexor is the most curative.
- Studies show that Wellbutrin, perhaps Serzone, and possibly Remeron have the fewest sexual side effects.
- The danger of seizures from Wellbutrin can be minimized through careful dosing.

Summary of Wellbutrin, Effexor, Serzone, and Remeron

The following table compares some of the main characteristics of Wellbutrin, Effexor, Serzone, and Remeron.

	Wellbutrin	Effexor	Serzone	Remeron
Mechanism of action	Unknown* Weak dopamine and norepinephrine reuptake inhibitor	Norepinephrine and serotonin reuptake inhibitor	Two actions on serotonin and norepinephrine reuptake inhibitor	Increases release of norepinephrine and serotonin
Dosage frequency	3 ×/day	2–3 ×/day	2–3 ×/day	1 ×/day
Total amount daily	225–450 mg	75–375 mg	200–600 mg	15–45 mg
Possible side effects				
Sexual dysfunction	No	Yes	No	No
Dizziness, sleepiness	No	No	Yes	Yes
Anxiety, agitation, insomnia	Yes	Yes	No	No
Seizures	Yes	No	No	No
Hypertension	No	Yes	No	No
Weight gain	No	No	No	Yes
Severe low WBC**	No	No	No	Yes

*The metabolism of Wellbutrin is not fully understood
**White blood cell count

- Hypertension, sexual dysfunction, and anxiety/insomnia are drawbacks of Effexor.
- Dizziness or feelings of weakness and lack of energy are problems with Serzone and Remeron, but they do not raise blood pressure (as does Effexor) and do not make people feel agitated and "wired" (as do all of the others).
- Remeron has the advantage of once-a-day dosage, but weight gain from it may be a drawback. I do not know how serious its rare effect on white blood cells will prove to be.

All of these four drugs have advantages over the SSRIs regarding activation (anxiety, insomnia) or sexual dysfunction, all but Remeron have the disadvantages of multiple dosing and of requiring close monitoring for dose elevation to achieve maximum efficacy, and each has a drawback: Wellbutrin may cause seizures, Effexor may raise blood pressure, Serzone and Remeron may cause dizziness or feelings of weakness and loss of energy. But more important than these side effect differences (in some cases, minor), the main drawback of all these new antidepressants as well as the old ones is that about 30 percent of people do not respond, and another 20 percent do so only partially, and are not completely cured. It is for these people who continue suffering that more effective treatments must be found. The next chapter is devoted to the treatment-resistant depressed individual.

CHAPTER 5

What If You're Still Depressed?

The new drugs make most depressed people feel like their old selves, and some who have been down for years feel better than they can ever remember. In this spirit of excitement and the hope that effective, safe relief from this painful affliction is now available, I am reluctant to temper enthusiasm with talk of failure. It is tempting to promise, as the ad in the psychiatric journals does, that Prozac will "restore the person within the patient," and much more dreary to add the qualifier that this is true in only 50 to 70 percent of cases. It is important that you know that if the initial treatment does not work for you or your loved one (although the chances are very good that it will), you should not lose hope, because there are many other helpful alternatives available.

You should be prepared for the fact that 40 (some say 50) percent of people fail to respond to the first antidepressant they try, whether it is an SSRI or any other. Of this group, half do not respond because the medication does not work, and the other half because of an inability to tolerate the side effects. This means that when and if you decide to begin antidepressant medication, you should do so with the hope that you will be helped, but not necessarily by the first drug. Rather than thinking there is one miracle drug that will cure you, it is better to have the attitude that there are a group of outstanding medications, one of which has a great chance of being effective, though which one that is may not be evident on the first try.

If you are able to tolerate the side effects of the first drug and have not responded fully after a month at full dosage, it makes sense to take stock of the following factors when deciding what to do:

1. If you feel a little better, then allow more time, and perhaps try a higher dosage (especially if it is a non-SSRI with a higher cure rate at bigger amounts). You probably will need another month or two on the same drug if you are able to stand the pain and can wait. Those with very severe symptoms may not have that luxury.
2. If you are severely ill, then it may take as much as six months before you feel normal on any drug. You should try to be patient until the medication works fully.
3. If you have not responded in the least at full dosage after several months, it is time to taper off the drug you are on (it is rarely advisable to stop suddenly) and prepare to go on another.

Trying Again

If you don't respond to the first drug tried or cannot tolerate it, it is advisable to try a second one. These days, most people receive an SSRI first. Many who stop because of side effects respond comfortably to a second SSRI. But those who can tolerate but do not get better on full dosage of a first SSRI may want to switch to a different kind of antidepressant. There haven't been any carefully controlled studies to determine whether a drug of a different family is more effective than another SSRI, but clinical lore favors Wellbutrin, Effexor, Serzone, and perhaps Remeron over a second SSRI. I know of individual cases in which a person responded to a second SSRI, and others where the non-SSRI worked. In any event, about half of the initial 40 to 50 percent of drug failures respond to the second drug. By this time, about 80 percent have significantly improved, although they may not be entirely well.

There are several groups of patients that seem to respond less well to the first drug tried. Elderly people can be less responsive, as can those with very severe symptoms, those with psychotic or bipolar depression, and those who have other psychiatric or medical conditions complicating their depression. In most clinical trials, these complicated cases are excluded before a new antidepressant is released. Thus, research subjects are usually fairly young (in their thirties and forties), do not have other psychiatric or medical illnesses, are not chronically depressed or suicidal, and are not taking other drugs. Once the FDA approves the medication, it is prescribed for the difficult, previously unresponsive person on whom it was never tested. The difference between the "easy" conditions for which the drug was originally given and the "hard" ones it must combat in the real world can easily be seen if one observes the placebo response in the prerelease subject and in the real one. In the former, it is 25 to 40 percent, whereas in the treatment-resistant patient, it is 0 to 10 percent. It takes a powerful drug to improve or cure treatment-resistant depression, not a sugar pill.

Treatment-Resistant Depression (TRD)

Twenty percent of people fail to improve on either the first or second drug tried. These people are called treatment-resistant. At this point, there are two options: adding another drug to the existing treatment or changing to a third drug. If, for example, Paxil failed first and Wellbutrin second, then one of the following drugs can be added to Wellbutrin:

Lithium
Thyroid (T$_3$)
A tricyclic
A stimulant

If these four alternatives (to be discussed in the following sections) fail, it is possible to turn at any time to the still most effective treatment of depression: electroshock therapy (see page 156).

The less proven second drug additions, which have no controlled but only anecdotal support, are:

Reserpine
Antipsychotic drugs
A high-dose MAOI
A tricyclic-and-MAOI combination
Yohimbine
An anticonvulsant
L-Tryptophan
Estrogen
Buspirone

Adding Lithium

Lithium is a naturally-occurring substance that is primarily used in treating manic-depressive illness. The addition of lithium is the most effective next step against TRD. Some people get better rapidly and dramatically, and others more slowly when lithium is added. Experience in combining lithium with the SSRIs is much more limited than with the tricyclics. The Prozac/lithium combination can be troubled by unpleasant side effects. After four weeks, over 50 percent of TRD patients improve following the addition of lithium.

Adding Thyroid (T₃)

L-triiodothyronine (T_3) is produced by the thyroid. It can also be administered in the form of a drug used for TRD. Added to the previously ineffective antidepressant, T_3 speeds the response of depressed women, but not men. Some believe that, in general, T_3 only works in women with borderline thyroid abnormalities rather than in depressed women (and men). It is generally thought that 25 to 50 percent of tricyclic-treated TRD patients improve when T_3 is added, and there is little toxicity risk in doing so. T_3 addition to the new antidepressants has not yet been adequately studied.

Combining a Tricyclic with an SSRI

Combination of the tricyclic desipramine with Prozac or some other SSRI seems to work well, but needs further controlled proof of its effectiveness. When Prozac or Paxil is the first drug tried, it must be remembered to keep the desipramine doses small (e.g., 50 mg) because of the effect of these two SSRIs on liver metabolism, while Zoloft presents less of an interaction worry.

Adding Ritalin or Dexedrine

Ritalin and Dexedrine are stimulants. There is no controlled research to support the practice of adding them to antidepressants, but one open study found that five of seven TRD patients improved rapidly and markedly with this combination. Pemoline (Cylert), another stimulant, can also be added instead of Ritalin or Dexedrine, and is easier to prescribe because it is not a class II controlled substance, and as such can be called in by the doctor to the pharmacist over the phone.

In my experience, an occasional TRD patient responds dramatically to the addition of up to 30 mg of Dexedrine or up to

60 mg of Ritalin without suffering side effects or ending up abusing the drug. People who drink a lot of coffee may do better, whereas those who cannot tolerate caffeine may not like a stimulant drug, but this is not an infallible predictor. Since it is not possible to know in advance who will benefit from the addition of a stimulant, it is worth a trial in the suffering TRD person.

People with TRD vary in their response to stimulants, from those who feel agitated and "wired," to those who initially feel better and then show no signs of improvement, to still others who respond well to a low dose and continue to do so for months or even years.

For the 10 to 15 percent who remain ill even after combinations of an antidepressant with lithium, thyroid, a tricyclic, and a stimulant, who are suffering and deeply discouraged, having difficulty working, and are a burden to themselves and their families, whose distress is severe and danger of suicide great, electroshock therapy should be considered.

Electroshock Therapy
(Electroconvulsive Therapy, or ECT)

If you have ever woken up with a hangover, you realize how susceptible your brain is to poison. In severe depression, the chemical changes are just as powerful, whether they are due to serotonin imbalance or, as the ancients thought, to "black bile." Unlike with a hangover, the misery of depression lasts for months. We do not know why certain depressions occur, but they can strike any of us, ruining our sleep, our ability to work and concentrate, and our interest in food, sex, and hobbies. Depression can also destroy our feelings of love and friendship, rob us of laughter, cause us to turn to alcohol for anesthesia, and make us feel completely alone in our misery. Furthermore, the reason for all this suffering may remain unknown, or the reasons offered by the patient or a family member may seem too trivial to be judged causal.

Psychiatrists would like to be able to point to verifiable causes of clearly defined diseases, but instead must list symptoms occurring together comprising syndromes which give the picture of illnesses, but whose origin is unknown. Electroshock therapy is a treatment in which a current of electricity is passed through the brain. It is not known exactly how or why it works to relieve depression, but it has been shown to be effective when all other treatments have failed. At first, the alternative of ECT may seem barbaric to the patient and concerned loved ones around him or her, and even to the physician, who may wonder whether he or she is reacting out of frustration at being unable to cure what can be an annoying, complaining person or a stoic who denies that anything is wrong, when so much obviously is. Perhaps the physician should try harder to understand, to listen more carefully to the patient's account of his or her pain, and to offer relief through empathy, thus sharing the burden of the distress. It is too easy for the helper to avoid the sufferer's need for a touch of humanity and turn out of haste and avoidance to the magic of electricity. There are bad doctors who have run "shock factories" in which ECT was given routinely, without thought or caring. But there are other kinds of bad doctors and therapists who wait too long while continuing ineffective psychotherapy and drugs for those in severe pain, 15 percent of whom commit suicide. The patient may reject help and maintain a falsely brave front while secretly preparing to terminate his life. The physician may have to urge, even force, electroshock on reluctant or resistant individuals who fear their brains will be fried and damaged and their memories destroyed. Some disturbed psychiatric patients are like people in a coma, in need of emergency treatment without being aware of it, and unless someone takes responsibility (the next of kin or legal conservator), such a person could commit suicide or die from starvation.

Modern ECT is not medieval torture or a form of barbarism. The anesthetist administers a muscle relaxant and oxygen, and puts the patient to sleep, allaying the fears of both the recipient and his or her relatives. Overall, dramatic relief occurs in over 80 percent of those treated, and in about 50 to 75 percent of the TRD patients. Those who have been helped by it return requesting ECT again when and if their depression recurs. They are often unwilling to wait for what they consider useless drug and psychotherapy trials, and want relief as rapidly as possible. The treatments do not necessarily require the patient to be hospitalized, only someone to drive them home afterward, and sometimes can be done while the person continues in his usual occupation. The electrodes can both be placed over the right cerebral hemisphere for a right-handed person (unilateral non-dominant) or on both sides of the head (bilateral). The modern use of unilateral (one-sided) ECT significantly decreases the problem of post-treatment amnesia, although bilateral administration is more effective and should be tried if unilateral ECT does not work.

Memory problems following ECT, whether one-sided or bilateral, are minimal. They are confined, when present, to information acquired shortly before ECT was given. Memory difficulties usually disappear completely within six months of treatment.

ECT is equal to, if not superior to, all other therapies used to treat severe TRD. About 50 to 75 percent of those who do not respond to tricyclics improve with ECT. Once the TRD patient recovers, it is necessary either to use drugs or to continue ECT to prevent recurrence. Some people, unfortunately, do not improve after a full course of twelve ECT treatments (including at least six bilateral ones). Following a brief medication-free period, a previously untried anti-depressant drug may be successful, perhaps because the ECT has somehow changed the sensitivity of the synapse.

Why Am I Still Depressed?

If you continue to be depressed after trying an antidepressant, there may be another factor contributing to your condition. These factors are:

Type of depression
Medical illnesses
Drugs causing depression
Complicating psychiatric illnesses
Demographic factors

Type of Depression

Some kinds of depression respond better to certain drugs than others do. The diagnosis of psychotic depression can be missed because the patients are ashamed and hide their delusion (a false fixed belief) that they are worthless and feel utter despair. When they are treated with an antidepressant drug alone, only 35 percent respond, whereas 70 percent of non-delusional depressives recover. When an antipsychotic is added to the antidepressant, there is a much higher recovery rate. If this fails, ECT may be necessary, and is most effective.

Atypical depressives (those whose moods are reactive to the environment and who sleep and eat too much) respond better to MAOIs (Nardil, Parnate) and sometimes to the new antidepressants. Bipolar patients without energy may do better on MAOIs and/or possibly on Wellbutrin and lithium.

Medical Illnesses Interfering with Depression Recovery

The following is a list of medical conditions that can cause depression or interfere with its cure. If you suffer from any of these, be sure to let your doctor know before an antidepressant is prescribed.

Anemia
Gastrointestinal disease (e.g., Crohn's disease)
Neurological diseases
   multiple sclerosis
   Parkinson's disease
   Huntington's disease
   dementia

    stroke
    brain tumors
Endocrine diseases
    thyroid
    pituitary
    adrenal
Infectious diseases
    hepatitis
    influenza
    AIDS
Lupus erythematosus
Heart disease
Malignancies

Drugs That Cause or Worsen Depression

Many drugs used to treat medical conditions may cause or worsen depression, making it more difficult to cure. If you are taking any of the following drugs, be sure to let your physician know before an antidepressant is prescribed.

    Drugs for high blood pressure
        Inderal (propranolol)
        Catapres (clonidine)
        Aldomet (methyldopa)
        reserpine
    Cortisone
    Hormones
        estrogen
        progesterone
    Anticancer drugs
        vincristine
        vinblastine
    Parkinson's disease drugs
        Sinemet, etc. (levodopa, carbidopa)
        amantadine

Simultaneous Psychiatric Conditions
Making Recovery More Difficult

If the factors just cited can be ruled out, then other psychiatric or personality disorders should be considered as reasons for why antidepressant drug therapy has failed. These so-called comorbid states (the simultaneous appearance of two or more illnesses, like depression and alcoholism, in which one may be causing the other, or both may be the product of some hidden factor) are evidence of the difficulty in clearly delineating psychiatric conditions. The hospital chart of a chronic patient almost never lists one pure illness, but a large number of psychiatric and personality disorders. Here are some of the disorders that impede recovery from depression:

Double Depression

People with lifelong dysthymia (chronic low-grade depression) are subject to superimposed major depressions, and after treatment may not fully recover but return to their chronic dysthymia.

Obsessive-Compulsive Disorder (OCD)

Sufferers of OCD also have frequent major depressive episodes. An antidepressant may relieve their depression, but not their OCD. OCD patients need higher doses of serotonergic antidepressants for many months in order for their OCD to improve. Unfortunately, many, while significantly helped, do not completely recover.

Panic Disorder

Panic disorder patients are prone to episodes of major depression, and major depressives are prone to panic attacks. A person with panic disorder who develops major depression recovers more slowly than someone with depression alone, and has a poorer response to antidepressants. Major depressives who are very anxious but do not suffer panic attacks are also slower in their response to medication. This does not mean you should be overly concerned about your panic disorder, but you should be prepared to wait a little longer until your antidepressant works.

Alcohol and Substance Abuse

More than a quarter of all depressives abuse alcohol or illicit drugs. Ongoing substance abuse in depressed people spoils their response to antidepressant medication. The alcohol or drug problem must be addressed separately and successfully controlled in order for the depression to be medicated and resolved.

Two self-administered tests for alcoholism are widely used: the CAGE and the MAST. The term CAGE refers to a device used to remember four questions: (1) Have you ever had to *c*ut down on alcohol? (2) Has anyone *a*nnoyed you with descriptions of how much you drink? (3) Have you felt *g*uilty about the quantity you consume? (4) Have you needed an *e*ye-opener to get going or relieve a hangover? The Michigan Alcoholism Screening Test (MAST) includes twenty-five items consisting of questions about the amount of drinking and alcohol-related, next-day memory loss, family complaints, fights, work interference, liver cirrhosis, DTs (delirium tremens), hospitalizations, and about morning drinking, drunk driving, and alcohol-related arrests.

When new antidepressant drugs are studied before FDA approval, they are tried on people who are *not* active substance abusers. The reason is that antidepressant drug failures are high among alcoholics and drug addicts. In one study of bipolar disorder, there were five times as many treatment failures in the abuse group as in the nonabuse group. If alcohol or drugs have made you depressed, or if you take them because you are depressed, you need to stop this self-injurious behavior in order for your antidepressant drug to work.

Eating Disorders

People with bulimia or anorexia nervosa and major depression do not respond very well to antidepressants alone, and require a combination of behavior therapy, group therapy, and nutritional guidance.

Personality Disorders

Personality disorders are defined by the *Diagnostic and Statistical Manual* (4th ed., 1994) as patterns of inflexible and maladaptive traits that cause subjective distress and significant impairment in social life and occupational functioning. These patterns are continually present since childhood or adolescence and influence

- awareness, perception, reasoning, and judgment
- the regulation of emotions
- control over impulses
- how needs are gratified
- how the person relates to others

People with personality disorders are inflexible, respond poorly to the changes and demands of life, and lack resilience. Most of them are unaware that their personality causes them problems, deny they have difficulties, and are quick to blame others. People with personality disorders have trouble with all aspects of their lives; they are likely to have stormy relationships, to be divorced, and to be fired from jobs. These adversities in their work, social, and intimate lives make them vulnerable to depression, and impede their recovery once they become ill.

There are three schools of thought about the relationship between personality disorder and depression: (1) Certain kinds of personalities lead to depression; (2) Suffering from depression changes personality; and (3) Personality and depression are both influenced by the same underlying genetic forces. There are ten personality disorders listed in the *DSM IV:*

The Odd Cluster	The Dramatic, Emotional, Erratic Cluster	The Anxious, Fearful Cluster
Paranoid	Antisocial	Avoidant
Schizoid	Borderline	Dependent
Schizotypal	Histrionic	Obsessive-Compulsive
	Narcissistic	

While depressive symptoms can occur in anyone with a personality disorder, they are most common in the dramatic and anxious clusters. The dramatic group are impulsive, their inhibitions toward action lowered, and their moods unstable, rapidly shifting in response to frustration or separation from the people who are important to them. Fifty percent of those with borderline personality disorder suffer significant depression, which does not respond well to antidepressant drugs. Borderline persons feel empty, lonely, needy, and angry. They are supersensitive to rejection, have stormy or nonexistent interpersonal relationships, and are subject to moods that are reactive, indeed too reactive, to the environment. SSRIs help borderlines, but more proof of their efficacy in treating this condition is needed. Long-term psychotherapy is essential in this group of individuals.

Assertive, independent, competitive people are more likely to respond to antidepressant drug treatment than are those who are dependent and seek the fulfillment of their needs through other people. Perhaps the latter group would do better on long-term psychotherapy.

A depressed person with medical, psychiatric, and personality complications can be helped by antidepressant medication, but the cure becomes more difficult. The other factors must be addressed and modified to aid the antidepressant in its therapeutic effect. The Greek philosopher Heraclitus said in the fifth century B.C. that "a man's character is his fate." If his character keeps destroying his family, intimacies, and work life, and leaves him vulnerable to depression, then the pill alone is not the answer.

Demographics of Depression

Demography is the study of the characteristics of a certain population. Nowhere is this study trickier than in depression, in which it is necessary to differentiate personality features and the severity and duration of the illness from factors such as age, sex, education, income, social supports, and marital and work status which seem to predict outcome. These factors, so-called demographics, can be nothing more than measurements of the severity and chronicity of the illness. For example, a chronically, seriously ill depressed woman has less energy and confidence to go out and meet men, and therefore is more likely to remain single. To say she is depressed because she is unmarried makes no sense. A person may be sick because of being unmarried or because of marital difficulty, or the individual may be single or in a bad marriage because of being sick. The psychiatric epidemiologist Myrna Weissman found a sixfold increase in marital and family trouble in major depressives. Another study found that women in unhappy marriages had a poorer prognosis for recovery from depression. Is this because depressed people do not get along well with their spouses and are unable to confide in them? While it may be difficult to determine whether the depression caused the marital discord or vice versa, it is clear that working to repair the marital relationship aids the depressed person. Drs. K. Daniel O'Leary and Steven Beach successfully treated thirty-six troubled marriages in which the wives were depressed, resulting in greater marital satisfaction and a significant reduction in depression. Sometimes the marital improvement follows upon the relief of depression rather than causes it. Karen, the forty-year-old married mother of one I mentioned in a previous chapter, whose husband was cold and angry at what he thought to be her laziness and lack of attention to him and their child, became much warmer when Prozac lifted her depression, helping her to get out of bed and look as though she liked, rather than hated, him. Karen's demographics improved because her depression got better.

As bad as marriage can be, depression has been found in epidemiological studies to be much higher among the non-married population. The onset of depression is most likely in single women. Divorce or separation increases the likelihood of a first depressive episode, and decreases the recovery rate once it occurs. But a person's marital status does not affect his or her response to antidepressant drugs.

A depressive is more likely to recover if friends and family are warm, loving, and supportive, and less so if they are critical and hostile. The problem is that sicker depressives frustrate their families more, making them angry and disparaging, while healthier ones are less annoying. Ironically, the more needy the patient, the more the loved ones are turned off. It is the doctor's role to help the critical spouse and angry family to deal with the depressed person in a kinder, more supportive manner, because no matter how powerful the antidepressant medication, it is usually too weak to work all by itself, and requires the help of a friendly family.

Paula Clayton, of Washington University in St. Louis, and her colleagues found that a close, confiding relationship and physical closeness protected people from depression. Other investigators have discovered that the absence of social supports increases the patient's vulnerability to depression. Since depression keeps people home, withdrawn from society, this may be simply one more measurement of severity. People too impaired to go out and build and maintain social supports may become depressed because they are too sick to socialize, making the finding a redundancy. It does no good to suggest to the depressed that they venture out and form meaningful relationships so they will feel better.

Negative life events decrease the rate of recovery on antidepressant drugs. While this seems obvious, it pays to remember that if you lose your job or your lover or develop a serious medical illness while being treated with Prozac for depression, your recovery will be slowed down.

Summary: Steps to Take If You or a Loved One Are Treatment-Resistant

1. Take an antidepressant that agrees with you (i.e., the side effects are bearable) for several months at the right dose. If there is some noticeable improvement, give it more time, perhaps six months or a year, until you fully recover. But if after several months you feel no better, taper off and then stop.

2. The second drug you take may, but probably should not, belong to the same class as the first. Follow an SSRI with Wellbutrin, Serzone, Effexor, Remeron, or a tricyclic.

3. If you remain symptomatic, ask your doctor to add lithium, thyroid (best if you are a woman), a tricyclic antidepressant, or a stimulant to the antidepressant you are currently taking.

4. If everything up to now has failed, and you or a loved one remains in severe pain and unable to function for over a year, a course of twelve ECT treatments (six bilateral ones) should be considered before more time elapses and the suffering, despair, and suicidal thoughts worsen. This seemingly barbaric treatment has been modernized and civilized, and can produce startling results in the carefully chosen person.

5. If you and your doctor decide to skip the ECT step because you are adamantly opposed to it or not incapacitated enough, there are a series of other drugs you can try whose efficacy has mostly anecdotal support, and sometimes a smattering of controlled, objective verification. They are:

Reserpine
Antipsychotics
An MAOI
An MAOI-tricyclic combination
An anticonvulsant
L-Tryptophan

Estrogen
Buspirone
Yohimbine

6. If you still continue to be depressed, review the original diagnosis carefully, making sure of the following: you do not have previously unsuspected psychotic depression; there is no unknown medical condition preventing recovery; other drugs you are taking are not making you depressed; and you do not have a simultaneous psychiatric illness or personality disorder preventing recovery.

The End of Depression

Depressed people experience their demographics as bad, and must convert the most important of them to good—working alone, in a support group, or with a friend, therapist, or member of the clergy.

Demographics, as I have defined them before, are the characteristics describing a group of people: their age, sex, education, marital status, occupation, income level, family size, community involvement, religious affiliation, leisure pursuits, etc. Think about these parts of your life and how you would rate them. Depressed people usually regard their demographics as miserable. The depressive's demographics are experienced as: age—too old; sex—the wrong one; education—defective; marriage—miserable; single—hopelessly so; job—unbearable; income—inadequate; family—childless, none, or too demanding; community involvement—none or too much; religion—none or dissatisfied with; and leisure activities—boring. Direct work on the demographics of the TRD's (treatment-resistance depressive's) life is absolutely necessary and can be very helpful. Somewhere in this list often lies the most important part of the depressive's life, which makes the rest unacceptable and is the reason why the person is resistant to all antidepressants, whether old, new, or yet to be released. If marital therapy can make some people less depressed, as has been shown, then finding out what an individual's most important issue is and helping him or her to change it from miserable to pleasurable can result in startling improvement. A partially working antidepressant can sometimes provide enough help so that the person can overcome that which has kept him or her depressed, but it is the demographic change which will convert the half-improved depressive to a cured one.

I remember several questions, all referring to this essential point of change from depression to a life of energy and pleasure, posed by two men of very different, yet similar occupations, for whom I have the greatest respect: the late Elvin Semrad, M.D., psychiatrist, psychoanalyst, and teacher, and Father John Padberg, S.J. Semrad's questions were asked of patients interviewed in front of psychiatrists in training, and Father John's were asked of me alone late one evening. These words may not make the most exciting reading, but pause and try to honestly answer them. Believe me, they are not easy.

What do you really care about?
Whom do you really care about?
What do you need to do for yourself to make your life better?
Why are you not doing it?

These questions do not allow the avoidance maneuver of the personality disorder sufferer, who blames his or her woes on others. Fix what you can fix and learn to accept and make the best of what you cannot. Go back and read the depressive demographics; make the best of those you cannot change and radically alter those you can. Do it alone or work with a therapist or someone else you trust, but start the job today of fixing your life for the better. It seems obvious to me that if after all the steps described in this chapter, you are still not cured, then the cure is meant to come not from outside people or medications but from within. Ask yourself what you need so as not to be depressed, and go get it.

CHAPTER 6

What Does the Future Hold?
Antidepressants Available in
Other Places or Being Developed
in the United States

When we attend a baseball game, an opera, or a play, the talk often turns to the young talent on the way up. The great ones are easy to spot—unhittable pitchers, blasting batters, soaring singers, enthralling actors. The enjoyment of discovering the new and exciting extends to every area: the latest chef, clothing designer, architect, physician, automobile, computer, presidential candidate. We all yearn for progress and perfection. Nowhere is that yearning stronger than in medicine—the wish to be freed from the misery of painful bodily illness, the horror of cancer and stroke, the broken mind of schizophrenia, and what many describe as the most painful and debilitating affliction of all, depression. Depression both destroys the pleasures of life and makes its inevitable pains completely unbearable. The normal sadness following an illness or death, business reversal, or social slight becomes weighed down by depression, which destroys resilience, the chance for recovery, and the ability to try again.

In this chapter, I will try to be your guide to the antidepressants that are not yet available or that are in development in the United States. Because these drugs are unavailable in the United States and we cannot go and see the production for ourselves, I will be very specific in describing the facts on which I base my reviews of these up-and-coming agents. There are enthusiastic and pessimistic reviewers—those who love the theater, and most of what they see in it, and those with lofty standards met only by John Gielgud and Laurence Olivier. An example of this is the differing views of two distinguished psychiatric professors about the new drugs I am about to describe. Dr. Leo Hollister, of the University of Texas, referred to the pace of development of new psychotherapeutic drugs as "glacial," noting that Prozac and Zoloft, although better tolerated and safer in overdose, are no more effective than antidepressants we have had for the past forty years. Of the new antidepressants in various stages of development, he finds none more effective than those already available. Dr. Carolyn Rabinowitz of George Washington University, on the other hand, is quoted in the July 1994 edition of *Psychiatric Times* on the "marvelous, unprecedented breakthroughs" in effective treatments for mental illness.

How New Drugs Get Released

The Food and Drug Administration is maddeningly slow. A typical drug takes nine years to journey from the beginning of human trials to a pharmacy. Prozac, for example, was created in 1972, clinical trials began in 1976, and the drug was released for marketing in 1988. This is typical. The average time from synthesis of an antidepressant to its release in the United States is fourteen years. Those fond of pointing out how many more drugs are available in Europe denounce our FDA for its excessive bureaucratic procedures, and a few have suggested privatizing the process to protect it from governmental delay. Others say many of the European drugs are marketed without adequate research support, and applaud American thoroughness. While I am sure the FDA could speed up the process without undue risk to the consumer, I also know of no European antidepressant that I would advise hopping on a plane to cross the Atlantic to buy.

There are three ways to find a new antidepressant. One is to give prospective agents to animals who have been placed in experimental environments designed for the screening of antidepressant drugs. A second, employing drug receptors in the brain to identify new compounds, is the most fashionably scientific, but so far has turned up copies of older agents, and no breakthroughs. Finally there is the creativity and intuition of alert, experienced clinicians who have, aided by luck, provided most of the advances in psychopharmacology: lithium, Thorazine, Tofranil, and the MAOIs. Using a new drug in an open trial, astute researchers are able to identify if it is effective, in what dosage, and for which patients. This open, non-blind method has been slighted in recent years in the rush to start formal random controlled trials. More prolonged and leisurely open study would decrease the number of copycat drugs and diminish the frequency of expensive, formally researched failures. The rigid, narrowly focused present system leads to antidepressants being released that have never been tried on typical office and hospitalized patients and have not been used long enough to see if they really work.

For every drug that is actually released in the United States, thousands are developed. Of those that are then tried on humans, only a quarter will eventually be approved for sale, after a period averaging about nine years. A new antidepressant will cost between $200 and $250 million to bring to market. These high development costs tend to inhibit innovation and provide one explanation for why new SSRIs are constantly being put forward, rather than an antidepressant that is truly novel. Rational drug design can become repetitive design.

Some Antidepressants Unavailable
in the United States

The search is on for antidepressants that are more effective, faster-acting, better tolerated, and safer in overdose than what is currently available. The last of these goals, regarding safety in overdose, seems already to have been achieved by the SSRIs, Serzone, Effexor, and perhaps, Remeron. The new drugs are pretty well tolerated, but there is room for improvement in the areas of gastrointestinal upset, agitation, insomnia, and sexual disturbance. But it is in the realm of efficacy and speed of action that the need for improvement is greatest, and in which not much progress has been made in forty years. None of the twenty-three drugs listed alphabetically in this section, some of which are available outside of the United States, are more effective or faster-acting than those currently available here. You need not lobby your congressional representative to get them released here sooner. What they may provide, however, are different modes of action in fighting depression, and research leads to future breakthroughs. Or perhaps we will have to continue to rely on serendipity. I would encourage doctors to keep their eyes open and not sit back passively in darkened rooms watching the slides of molecular biologists for the answer. I would also encourage their patients to keep telling them what works and what does not, so that the two, doctor and patient, can join in the hunt together. It is a hunt not only for the right drug but for the way to overcome depression, something that in most cases takes much more than a pill.

Some of the descriptions of these twenty-three drugs will be much longer than others, either because more is known or because the drugs seem to have more promise.

Adinazolam

Available in Europe, this is a benzodiazepine belonging to

the same overall family as Valium, and to the same benzodiazepine subfamily as Xanax and Klonopin. In a slow-release
preparation, it may be effective in treating panic disorder, but
the FDA advisory panel recommended against its approval for
this use. When taken over time, it apparently sensitizes neu-
rons to serotonin, which may make it worth trying in the treatment of depression. In a four-week trial comparing Elavil,
Valium, and Adinazolam in depression, Elavil was best, Valium
worst, and Adinazolam in the middle.

Adrafinil

This drug is available in France and is said to be effective in
treating depression, especially in those whose thinking is
impaired. It is believed to work by affecting norepinephrine
in the synapse.

Amineptine

Used as an antidepressant in France and several other
European and South American countries, it seems to be
equal to established antidepressants in efficacy. The research
supporting this claim is sparse: only one study included a
placebo group. Amineptine has stimulant action and possible
abuse potential. It acts on dopamine, and perhaps on norepinephrine and serotonin as well.

Brofaromine

This is a reversible inhibitor of monoamine oxidase-A
(RIMA) whose clinical trials have been discontinued by Ciba-
Geigy because its effectiveness seemed doubtful. This class of
drugs is discussed under Moclobemide, a RIMA whose clinical
trials continue.

Buspirone

Buspirone, gepirone, ipsapirone, and flesinoxan together constitute a family of drugs known as agonists to the $5HT_{1A}$ receptor. There are at least twelve different subtypes of serotonin receptors located pre- and postsynaptically in the brain and $5HT_{1A}$ is one of them.

Buspirone (Buspar) is available in the United States for the treatment of anxiety. The other three members of this class are in various stages of trial and may be released here within the next few years. The advantage of Buspar over the benzodiazepines like Valium and Xanax is that it produces very little sedation, abuse, or withdrawal difficulties. Because of its short metabolism, it must be taken three times a day. Unlike the benzodiazepines, Buspar does not produce an immediate effect. In fact, the complete response may take two to four weeks, which is explained by the need to desensitize the receptor ($5HT_{1A}$), which takes time. People who have had benzodiazepines in the past do not like Buspar, because its action is too slow, there is no immediate mild euphoria, and there is no sedating effect. Nervous, anxious people like to be calmed now, not three weeks later. The main side effects of Buspar are headaches, restlessness, insomnia, nausea, and dizziness, a lineup that sounds suspiciously like that of an SSRI. The drug is safe in overdose.

Captopril (Capoten)

This drug is available in the United States as an antihypertensive. It is an angiotensin-converting enzyme (ACE) inhibitor, and has been reported to have mood-elevating effect in some patients. No controlled clinical trials of depressed patients have been published.

Citalopram

Citalopram is an SSRI available in Denmark and Sweden, with a number of controlled studies finding it effective. It probably will not be approved in the United States because of possible toxicity in primates identified in one study. I can find no other references to this toxicity. It is possible that the company decided the United States did not need yet another SSRI or there were patent problems (not enough time left before it became generic and less profitable). The drug can be taken once a day in doses of 40 to 60 mg, and as with the other SSRIs, its main side effect is nausea.

Dothiepin (Prothiaden)

Marketed elsewhere in the world, this drug is very similar to doxepin (Sinequan, Adapin, etc.), an older tricyclic available here with a lot of tricyclic-like side effects.

Duloxetine

This drug is undergoing clinical trials for release in the United States and seems to act in the same fashion as Effexor—namely, it specifically inhibits the reuptake of both norepinephrine and serotonin without causing all the unwanted side effects of Elavil and the older tricyclics. While the notion of double, rather than single, action is pleasing to the mind (and perhaps the advertiser), it does not seem to produce a higher cure rate. I hope duloxetine is more than a "me, too" Effexor, and await proof of its greater efficacy.

Fengabine

The neurotransmitter gamma-aminobutyric acid (GABA) is involved in anxiety, and its effect is aided by benzodiazepines like Valium. GABA is also involved in the modulation of mood. Drugs that mimic GABA may be useful antidepressants. Fengabine has had antidepressant effects on patients (as has a similar drug, Progabide). No one seems too excited about these drugs as antidepressants, and I can find no signs of current clinical trials.

Idazoxan

The theory underlying this drug is that it acts by increasing norepinephrine in the synaptic cleft, and therefore should be an antidepressant. The controlled trials said to have been conducted on this drug have yet to be published. Let us hope it works.

Lofepramine

This tricyclic antidepressant is popular in the United Kingdom because it is said to be safe in overdosage and low in side effects. It is superior to a placebo and comparable to other antidepressants. Curiously, its major metabolite is desipramine (Norpramin), a drug we already have plenty of, so I doubt that lofepramine will ever be released here.

Mianserin (Bolvidon, Norval)

This older tetracyclic is probably a little less effective than standard antidepressants, as shown in double-blind studies. In use since 1976, it has never been available in the United States and no one misses it. It is available in five European countries. What interests researchers about mianserin is that it functions a little like Serzone on the serotonin receptor, and a little like idazoxan on the norepinephrine system.

Medifoxamine

This drug inhibits dopamine reuptake, as does the previously discussed amineptine, and is also available in France. There is only one published report of its antidepressant efficacy.

Minaprine

At 400 mg a day, minaprine is a well-tolerated and effective antidepressant which may also improve memory. The drug does not seem to be a stimulant or subject to abuse, and its main side effects are insomnia, anxiety, and nausea.

Moclobemide

The conventional MAOIs Nardil and Parnate irreversibly inhibit monoamine oxidase, thus raising the amounts of norepinephrine and serotonin in the synapse. When their use is discontinued, the body requires two weeks before it can produce the natural enzyme monoamine oxidase again. The danger of severe, life-threatening high blood pressure and of the serotonin syndrome (in its worst form producing high fever, circulatory failure, and death) limits the use of these drugs, and requires that careful dietary and medication restrictions be imposed.

The new MAOIs are reversible in their inhibition of monoamine oxidase in the hope that their side effects and dangers, and the dietary restrictions they necessitate, will be much less. Moclobemide is a reversible inhibitor of MAO-A (only the A form is required for antidepressant activity). The class to which it belongs is abbreviated as RIMA (reversible inhibitor monoamine oxidase-A). It is available in Canada and the United Kingdom, and has been used by some investigators for many years. The chance of severe hypertension occurring due to eating certain foods with the drug is reported to be very rare, although caution is advised when combining it with SSRIs or opioids. The dose range is 300 to 900 mg per day. In the United States, it is in clinical trial for panic disorder and social phobia, but not for depression. It has a half-life of only two hours.

There are reports that Moclobemide causes irritability, insomnia, anxiety, restlessness, and agitation. Some have found it not to be as effective as Nardil or Parnate. When taken alone in overdose, it is usually not fatal, but causes fatigue, agitation, and high blood pressure. In overdose and combined with other drugs, it can cause coma, high fever, rigidity, and even higher blood pressure, and when overdose of a RIMA is combined with an SSRI or the serotonin tricyclic Anafranil, the result can be lethal. Five deaths from this combination have been reported in Finland. Other RIMA dangers occur when these drugs are mixed with Demerol or nasal decongestants. The picture of the RIMAs continues to sharpen in focus, and does not appear as bright as it once was. We will have to keep watching to see if Moclobemide will be approved for use in the United States.

Modafanil

This drug is used in France for depression, although there is no published evidence of its antidepressant efficacy. It is believed to work through the norepinephrine system, and has psychostimulant properties.

Ondansetron (Zofran)

This drug affects serotonin and is currently available in the United States as an antiemetic agent for those undergoing chemotherapy, and to prevent postoperative nausea. Animal and human studies suggest that it may possess antianxiety, antidepressive, antipsychotic, antipanic, and anti–social phobic effects.

Ritanserin (Tisterton)

This drug has serotonin action similar to that of Serzone ($5HT_{2A}$ antagonist) and mianserin, and has promise of being an effective antidepressant. It is said to work in dysthymic and anxiety disorder patients as well. The drug is fairly far along in American clinical trials.

Roxindole

Roxindole acts on dopamine and on serotonin, which accounts for its antidepressant effects as well as for its ability to decrease depression and lack of energy in schizophrenics. It is not quite clear just what Roxindole does to dopamine (whether it increases or decreases it), but it seems to have antidepressant activity. It is in active clinical trial as an antidepressant in the United States.

S-Adenosyl-L-Methionine (SAMe)

This drug is thought to help brain cells manufacture neurotransmitters. Rapid antidepressant effects follow its intravenous administration, and several double-blind studies confirm its rapid action with few side effects. An oral form has been developed and has proved effective in a non-placebo-controlled trial. More research is obviously needed. Adding it to Tofranil in one study speeded the antidepressant response.

Sulpride (Dogmatil)

Sulpride has been used as an antipsychotic in Europe for years, and is also officially recognized in low doses as an antidepressant in France. There are no plans for its release in the United States.

Tianeptine

The unusual and interesting thing about this drug is that it is the opposite of an SSRI, which means it enhances rather than inhibits serotonin reuptake from the synapse. I mentioned this reduction of the intrasynaptic concentration of serotonin earlier, when I referred to kicking the synapse. If there is an explanation for what is happening in the gap between brain cells, it remains to be discovered.

Tianeptine is officially available only in France. The drug needs more research. In one controlled study of 265 anxious, dysthymic patients, Tianeptine was as effective as Elavil. In a published report on depressed alcoholics, it also equaled Elavil.

Tianeptine has no cardiovascular or older tricyclic-like side effects. Its most common side effects are vomiting, nausea, irritability, anxiety, and insomnia. There are currently no plans to release it in the United States.

What to Do Until
the Next Antidepressant Breakthrough

There you have it—the twenty-three drugs I have chosen to mention, some serious contenders for release in the United States, others theoretically interesting, some so you will know what your friends and relatives abroad are taking. I have chosen to leave out many others because they seem weak, toxic, or dull copies of what we already have. I am reminded of how forty years ago the great Swiss psychiatrist Roland Kuhn, working with a slightly modified form of Thorazine, which he expected to be an antipsychotic, had the clarity of vision to observe what he did not expect to see, and thus found Tofranil, the first tricyclic antidepressant. With all our progress, no antidepressant has proven more effective than this first one. It is clear that our diagnostic tools still need to be refined, as do the medications we use to treat what we diagnose. Many dedicated psychiatric researchers are occupied in doing just that.

But until the next significant breakthrough, depression sufferers have the eight presently available modern antidepressants described in this book. If you are truly lucky, they will completely cure you. If, like most patients, you are complicated and not totally cured, you at least have a chance of receiving some very good help in your efforts to get control of your feelings and your life, so that you will be able to function in a full and meaningful way. Who knows what miracle medication will come along next year, genetically engineered to root out the elusive depressive gene. Somehow I suspect humans do not work that way, and that our machine requires more than a drug. It requires love and useful activity of which we can be proud, and the identification of something worth living for. It takes more than Prozac to make a full life.

Bibliography

Depression and Its Treatment

Akiskal, H. S. 1984. The interface of chronic depression with personality and anxiety disorders. *Psychopharmocology Bulletin* 20:393–98.

American Psychiatric Association. Practice guideline for major depressive disorder in adults. 1993. *American Journal of Psychiatry* 150 (No. 4, suppl.).

Brown, W. A., and Harrison, W. 1995. Are patients who are intolerant to one selective serotonin reuptake inhibitor intolerant to another? *Journal of Clinical Psychiatry* 56: 30–34.

Coryell, W., Scheftner, W., Keller, M., et al. 1993. The enduring psychosocial consequences of mania and depression. *American Journal of Psychiatry* 150:720–27.

The Cross-National Collaborative Group. 1992. The changing rate of major depression. *JAMA* 268:3098–3105.

DeVane, C. L. 1994. Pharmacogenetics and drug metabolism of newer antidepressant agents. *Journal of Clinical Psychiatry* 55 (12, suppl.): 38–45.

Donovan, S. J., and Roose, S. P. 1995. Medication use during psychoanalysis: A survey. *Journal of Clinical Psychiatry* 56:177–78.

Dubovsky, S. L., and Thomas, M. 1995. Serotonergic mechanisms and current and future psychiatric practice. *Journal of Clinical Psychiatry* 56 (suppl. 2): 38–48.

Hays, R. D., Wells, K. B., Sherbourne, D. C., et al. 1995. Functioning and well-being outcomes of patients with depression compared with chronic medical illness. *Archives of General Psychiatry* 52:11–19.

Hirschfeld, R. M. A. 1994. Guidelines for the long-term treatment of depression. *Journal of Clinical Psychiatry* 55 (12, suppl.): 61–69.

Judd, L. L. 1994. Social phobia: A clinical overview. *Journal of Clinical Psychiatry* 55 (6, suppl.): 5–9.

Keller, M. B., and Hanks, D. L. 1994. The natural history and heterogeneity of depressive disorders: Implications for rational antidepressant therapy. *Journal of Clinical Psychiatry* 55 (9, suppl. A): 25–31.

———, Klerman, G. L., Lavori, P. W., et al. 1982. Treatment received by depressed patients. *JAMA* 248:1848–55.

———, Lavori, P. W., Mueller, T. I., et al. 1992. Time to recovery, chronicity, and levels of psychopathology in major depression. *Archives of General Psychiatry* 49:809–16.

Kocsis, J. H., Croughan, J. L., Katz, M. M., et al. 1990. Response to treatment with antidepressants of patients with severe or moderate nonpsychotic depression and of patients with psychotic depression. *American Journal of Psychiatry* 147:621–24.

Kupfer, D. J. 1993. Management of recurrent depressions. *Journal of Clinical Psychiatry* 54 (2, suppl.): 29–33.

———, Frank, E., Perel, J. M., et al. 1992. Five-year outcome for maintenance therapies in recurrent depression. *Archives of General Psychiatry* 49:769–73.

Leonard, B. E. 1993. The comparative pharmacology of new anti-depressants. *Journal of Clinical Psychiatry* 54 (suppl.): 3–15.

Liebowitz, M. R. 1989. Antidepressants in panic disorders. *British Journal of Psychiatry* 155 (suppl.): 46–52.

McTavish, D., and Benfield, P. 1990. Clomipramine: An overview of its pharmacological properties and a review of its therapeutic use in obsessive-compulsive disorder and panic disorder. *Drugs* 39:136–53.

Nemeroff, C. B. 1994. Evolutionary trends in the pharmacotherapeutic management of depression. *Journal of Clinical Psychiatry* 55 (12, suppl.): 3–15.

Preskorn, S. H. 1994. Antidepressant drug selection: Criteria and options. *Journal of Clinical Psychiatry* 55 (9, suppl. A): 6–22.

———. 1993. Pharmacokinetics of antidepressants: Why and how they are relevant to treatment. *Journal of Clinical Psychiatry* 54 (9, suppl.): 14–34.

———, and Burke, M. 1992. Somatic therapy for major depressive disorder: Selection of an antidepressant. *Journal of Clinical Psychiatry* 53 (9, suppl.): 5–18.

Regier, D. A., Hirschfield, R. M. A., Goodwin, F. K., et al. 1988. The NIMH depression awareness, recognition, and treatment program: Structure, aims, and scientific basis. *American Journal of Psychiatry* 145:1351–57.

Weinberger, D. R. 1993. SPECT imaging in psychiatry: Introduction and overview. *Journal of Clinical Psychiatry* 54 (11, suppl.): 3–5.

Weissman, M. M., Prusoff, B. A., Dimascio, A., et al. 1979. The efficacy of drugs and psychotherapy in the treatment of acute depressive episodes. *American Journal of Psychiatry* 136: 555–58.

Wells, K. B., Stewart, A. S., Hays, R. D., et al. 1989. The functioning and well-being of depressed patients. *JAMA* 262:914–19.

Fluoxetine (Prozac)

Bowden, C. L., Schatzberg, A. F., Rosenbaum, A., et al. 1993. Fluoxetine and desipramine in major depressive disorder. *Journal of Clinical Psychopharmacology* 13:305–10.

Fava, M., Rappe, S. M., Pava, J. A., et al. 1995. Relapse in patients on long-term fluoxetine treatment: Response to increased fluoxetine dose. *Journal of Clinical Psychiatry* 56:52–55.

————, and Rosenbaum, J. F. 1991. Suicidality and fluoxetine: Is there a relationship? *Journal of Clinical Psychiatry* 52:108–111.

Fluoxetine—a new specific serotonin reuptake inhibitor in major depressive disorder. 1985. *Journal of Clinical Psychiatry* 46 (3, sec. 2).

Gram, L. F. 1994. Fluoxetine. *New England Journal of Medicine* 17:1354–1361.

Kramer, P. D. 1993. *Listening to Prozac.* New York: Viking.

Montgomery, S. A., Dufour, H., Brion, S., et al. 1988. The prophylactic efficacy of fluoxetine in unipolar depression. *British Journal of Psychiatry* 153 (suppl. 3): 69–76.

Pande, A., and Sayler, M. 1993. Severity of depression and response to fluoxetine. *International Clinical Psychopharmocology* 8:243–45.

Pearlstein, T. B., and Stone, A. B. 1994. Long-term fluoxetine treatment of late luteal phase dysphoric disorder. *Journal of Clinical Psychiatry* 55:332–35.

Pigott, T. A., Pato, M. T., Bernstein, S. E., et al. 1990. Controlled comparisons of clomipramine and fluoxetine in the treatment of obsessive-compulsive disorder. *Archives of General Psychiatry* 47:926–32.

Rickels, K., Amsterdam, J. D., and Avallone, M. F. 1986. Fluoxetine in major depression: A controlled study. *Current Therapeutic Research* 39:559–63.

Roose, S. P., Glassman, A. H., Attia, E., et al. 1994. Comparative efficacy of selective serotonin reuptake inhibitors and tricyclics in the treatment of mania. *American Journal of Psychiatry* 151:1735–39.

Salzman, C., Wolfson, A. N., Schatzberg, A., et al. 1995. Effect of fluoxetine on anger in symptomatic volunteers with borderline personality disorder. *Journal of Clinical Psychopharmacology* 15:23–29.

Stone, A. B., Pearlstein, T. B., and Brown, W. A. 1991. Fluoxetine in
the treatment of late luteal phase dysphoric disorder. *Journal of
Clinical Psychiatry* 52:290–93.

Wernicke, J. F., Dunlop, S. R., Dornseif, B. E., et al. 1987. Fixed-dose
fluoxetine therapy for depression. *Psychopharmacology Bulletin*
23:164–68.

Sertraline (Zoloft)

Aguglia, E., Casacchia, M., Cassano, G. B., et al. 1993. Double-blind
study of the efficacy and safety of sertraline and fluoxetine
[Prozac] in major depression. *International Clinical Psychopharmacology* 8:197–202.

Bennie, E. H., Mullin, J. M., and Martindale, J. J. 1995. A double-
blind multicenter trial comparing sertraline and fluoxetine in
outpatients with major depression. *Journal of Clinical Psychiatry*
56:229–37.

Chouinard, G. 1992. Sertraline in the treatment of obsessive compulsive disorder: two double-blind, placebo-controlled studies.
International Clinical Psychopharmacology 7 (2, suppl.): 37–41.

Cole, J. O. 1992. New directions in antidepressant therapy: A review
of sertraline, a unique serotonin reuptake inhibitor. *Journal of
Clinical Psychiatry* 53:333–40.

Doogan, D. P., and Caillard, V. 1992. Sertraline in the prevention of
depression. *British Journal of Psychiatry* 160:217–22.

Fisher, S., Kent, T., and Bryant, S. 1995. Postmarketing surveillance
by patient self-monitoring: Preliminary data for sertraline versus
fluoxetine [Prozac]. *Journal of Clinical Psychiatry* 56:288–96.

Murdoch, D., and McTavish, D. 1992. Sertraline: A review of its
pharmacodynamic and pharmacokinetic properties and therapeutic potential in depression and obsessive-compulsive disorder.
Drugs 44:604–24.

Reimherr, F. W., Chouinard, G., Cohn, C. K., et al. 1990. Antidepressant efficacy of sertraline: A double-blind placebo and amitriptyline-controlled, multicenter comparison study in outpatients with major depression. *Journal of Clinical Psychiatry* 51 (12, suppl. B): 18–27.

Paroxetine (Paxil)

Ayd, F. J. 1993. Paroxetine: A new selective serotonin reuptake inhibitor. *International Drug Therapy Newsletter* 28 (2): 5–12.

Claghorn, J. L. 1992. The safety and efficacy of paroxetine compared with placebo in a double-blind trial of depressed outpatients. *Journal of Clinical Psychiatry* 53 (2, suppl.): 33–35.

Cohn, J. B., and Wilcox, C. S. 1992. Paroxetine in major depression: A double-blind trial with imipramine and placebo. *Journal of Clinical Psychiatry* 53 (2, suppl.): 52–56.

De Wilde, J., Spiers, R., Mertens, C., et al. 1993. A double-blind, comparative, multicentre study comparing paroxetine with fluoxetine in depressed patients. *Acta Psychiatrica Scandinavica* 87:141–45.

Dunbar, G. C., Cohn, J. B., Fabre, L. F., et al. 1991. A comparison of paroxetine, imipramine [Tofranil], and placebo in depressed out-patients. *British Journal of Psychiatry* 159:394–98.

Eric, L. 1991. A prospective, double-blind, comparative, multicentre study of paroxetine and placebo in preventing recurrent major depressive episodes [abstract]. *Biological Psychiatry* 29 (11 S): 254S–55S.

Fabre, L. F. 1992. A six-week, double-blind trial of paroxetine, imipramine, and placebo in depressed outpatients. *Journal of Clinical Psychiatry* 53 (2, suppl.): 40–43.

Feighner, J. P., and Boyer, W. F. 1992. Paroxetine in the treatment of depression: A comparison with imipramine and placebo. *Journal of Clinical Psychiatry* (2, suppl.): 44–47.

Kiev, A. 1992. A double-blind, placebo-controlled study of paroxetine in depressed outpatients. *Journal of Clinical Psychiatry* 53 (suppl.): 27–29.

Kreider, M. S., Bushnell, W. D., Oakes, R., et al. 1995. A double-blind, randomized study to provide safety information on switching fluoxetine-treated patients to paroxetine without an intervening washout period. *Journal of Clinical Psychiatry* 56:142–45.

Nemeroff, C. B. 1993. Paroxetine: An overview of the efficacy and safety of a new selective serotonin reuptake inhibitor in the treatment of depression. *Journal of Clinical Psychopharmacology* 13 (6, suppl. 2): 10S–17S.

Rickels, K., Amsterdam, J., Clary, C., et al. 1992. The efficacy and safety of paroxetine compared with placebo in outpatients with major depression. *Journal of Clinical Psychiatry* 53 (2, suppl.): 30–32.

Shrivastava, R. K., Shrivastava, S. H. P., Overweg, N., et al. 1992. A double-blind comparison of paroxetine, imipramine, and placebo in major depression. *Journal of Clinical Psychiatry* 53 (2, suppl.): 48–51.

Smith, W. T., and Glaudin, V. 1992. A placebo-controlled trial of paroxetine in the treatment of major depression. *Journal of Clinical Psychiatry* 53: (2, suppl.): 36–39.

Stuppaeck, C. H., Geretsegger, C., and Whitworth, A. B. 1994. A multicenter double-blind trial of paroxetine versus amitriptyline in depressed outpatients. *Journal of Clinical Psychopharmacology* 14:241–46.

Tignol, J. 1993. A double-blind, randomized, fluoxetine-controlled, multicenter study of paroxetine in the treatment of depression. *Journal of Clinical Psychopharmacology* 13 (6, suppl. 2): 18S–22S.

Fluvoxamine (Luvox)

Benfield, P., and Ward, A. 1986. Fluvoxamine: A review of its pharmacodynamic and pharmacokinetic properties and therapeutic efficacy in depressive illness. *Drugs* 32:313–34.

Burton, S. W. 1991. A review of fluvoxamine and its uses in depression. *International Clinical Psychopharmacology* (suppl. 3): 1–17; discussion, 17–21.

Conti, L., Dell'osso, L., Re, F., et al. 1988. Fluvoxamine maleate: Double-blind clinical trial vs. placebo in hospitalized depressed patients. *Current Therapeutic Research* 43:468–80.

McDougle, C. J., Goodman, W. K., Leckman, J. F., et al. 1993. The efficacy of fluvoxamine in obsessive-compulsive disorder: Effects of comorbid chronic tic disorder. *Journal of Clinical Psychopharmacology* 13:354–58.

Mendlewicz, J. 1992. Efficacy of fluvoxamine in severe depression. *Drugs* 43 (suppl. 2): 32–37; discussion, 37–39.

Montgomery, S. A., and Manceaux, A. 1992. Fluvoxamine in the treatment of obsessive-compulsive disorder. *International Clinical Psychopharmacology* (suppl. 1): 5–9.

Wilde, M. I., Plosker, G. L., and Benfield, P. 1993. Fluvoxamine: An updated review of its pharmacology and therapeutic use in depressive illness. *Drugs* 46 (5): 895–924.

Bupropion (Wellbutrin)

Clinical management of depression: Bupropion: An update. 1993. *Journal of Clinical Psychiatry*, monograph 11 (1).

Davidson, J. 1989. Seizures and bupropion: A review. *Journal of Clinical Psychiatry* 50:256–61.

Feighner, J. P., Gardner, E. A., Johnston, J. A., et al. 1991. Double-blind comparison of bupropion and fluoxetine [Prozac] in depressed outpatients. *Journal of Clinical Psychiatry* 52:329–35.

Gardner, E. A., and Johnston, J. A. 1985. Bupropion: An antidepressant without sexual pathophysiological action. *Journal of Clinical Psychopharmacology* 5:24–29.

Mendels, J., Amin, M. M., Chouinard, G., et al. 1983. A comparative study of bupropion and amitriptyline in depressed outpatients. *Journal of Clinical Psychiatry* 44:118–20.

Merideth, C. H., and Feighner, J. P. 1983. The use of bupropion in hospitalized depressed patients. *Journal of Clinical Psychiatry* 44:85–87.

Pitts, W. M., Fann, W. E., Halaris, A. E., et al. 1983. Bupropion in depression: A tricenter placebo-controlled study. *Journal of Clinical Psychiatry* 44:95–100.

Preskorn, S. H. 1991. Should bupropion dosage be adjusted based upon therapeutic drug monitoring? *Psychopharmacology Bulletin* 27:637–43.

Walker, P. W., Cole, J. O., Gardner, E. A., et al. 1993. Improvement in fluoxetine-associated sexual dysfunction in patients switched to bupropion. *Journal of Clinical Psychiatry* 54:459–65.

Weisler, R. H., Johnston, J. A., Lineberry, C. G., et al. 1994. Comparison of bupropion and trazodone for the treatment of major depression. *Journal of Clinical Psychopharmacology* 14:170–79.

Zarate, C. A., Tohen, M., Baraibar, G., et al. 1995. Prescribing trends of antidepressants in bipolar depression. *Journal of Clinical Psychiatry* 56:260–64.

Venlafaxine (Effexor)

Clerc, G. E., Ruimy, P., and Verdeau-Pailles, J. 1994. A double-blind comparison of venlafaxine and fluoxetine [Prozac] in patients hospitalized for major depression and melancholia. *International Clinical Psychopharmacology* 9:139–43.

Cunningham, L. A., Borison, R. L., Carman, J. S., et al. 1994. A comparison of venlafaxine, trazodone, and placebo in major depression. *Journal of Clinical Psychopharmacology* 14:99–106.

Derivan, A., Entsuah, R., Rudolph, R., et al. Early response to venlafaxine hydrochloride, a novel antidepressant. Proceedings of the 145th annual meeting of the American Psychiatric Association, May 2–7, 1992, Washington, D.C., pp. 82–83.

Feighner, J. P. 1994. The role of venlafaxine in rational antidepressant therapy. *Journal of Clinical Psychiatry* 55 (9, suppl. A): 62–68.

Guelfi, J. D., White, C., Hackett, D., et al. 1995. Effectiveness of venlafaxine in patients hospitalized for major depression and melancholia. *Journal of Clinical Psychiatry* 56:450–58.

Khan, A., Fabre, L. F., and Rudolph, R. R. 1991. Venlafaxine in
depressed outpatients. *Psychopharmacology Bulletin* 27 (2): 141–44.

Mendels, J., Johnston, R., Mattes, J., et al. 1993. Efficacy and safety
of b.i.d. [twice-daily] doses of venlafaxine in a dose-response
study. *Psychopharmacology Bulletin* 29 (2): 169–74.

Montgomery, S.A. 1993. Venlafaxine: A new dimension in antidepressant pharmacotherapy. *Journal of Clinical Psychiatry* 54:
119–26.

Nierenberg, A. A., Feighner, J. P., Rudolph, R. R., et al. 1994. Venlafaxine for treatment-resistant depression. *Neuropsychopharma-
cology* 10 (pt. 2): 85S.

Schweizer, E., Feighner, J., Mandos, L. A., et al. 1994. Comparison
of venlafaxine and imipramine in the acute treatment of major
depression in outpatients. *Journal of Clinical Psychiatry* 55: 104–8.

———, Weise, C., Clary, C., et al. 1991. Placebo-controlled trial
of venlafaxine for the treatment of major depression. *Journal of
Clinical Psychopharmacology* 11 (4): 233–36.

Shrivastava, R. K., Cohn, C., Crowder, J., et al. 1994. Long-term
safety and clinical acceptability of venlafaxine and imipramine
[Tofranil] in outpatients with major depression. *Journal of Clinical
Psychopharmacology* 14: 322–29.

The Venlafaxine French Inpatient Study Group. Clerc, G. E., et al.
1994. A double-blind comparison of venlafaxine and fluoxetine
in patients hospitalized for major depression and melancholia.
International Clinical Psychopharmacology 9 (3): 139–43.

Nefazodone (Serzone)

Anton, S., Robinson, D., Roberts, D., et al. 1994. Long-term treatment with nefazodone. *Psychopharmacology Bulletin* 30:165–69.

Feighner, J. P., Pambakian, R., Fowler, R. C., et al. 1989. A comparison of nefazodone, imipramine, and placebo in patients with moderate to severe depression. *Psychopharmacology Bulletin* 25:219–21.

Fontaine, R., Ontiveros, A., Elie, R., et al. 1994. A double-blind comparison of nefazodone, imipramine, and placebo in major depression. *Journal of Clinical Psychiatry* 55:234–41.

————, Ontiveros, A., Faludi, G., et al. 1991. A study of nefazodone, imipramine, and placebo in depressed outpatients. *Biological Psychiatry* 29:3–38.

Preskorn, S. H. 1995. Comparison of the tolerability of bupropion [Wellbutrin], fluoxetine [Prozac], imipramine [Tofranil], nefazodone [Serzone], paroxetine [Paxil], sertraline [Zoloft], and venlafaxine [Effexor]. *Journal of Clinical Psychiatry* 56 (suppl. 6): 12–21.

Rickels, K., Robinson, D. S., Schweizer, E., et al. 1995. Nefazodone: Aspects of efficacy. *Journal of Clinical Psychiatry* 56 (suppl. 6): 43–46.

————, Schweizer, E., Clary, C., et al. 1994. Nefazodone and imipramine in major depression: A placebo-controlled trial. *British Journal of Psychiatry* 164:802–5.

Sharpley, A. L., Walsh, A. E. S., Cowen, P. J. 1992. Nefazodone—a novel antidepressant—may increase REM sleep. *Biological Psychiatry* 31:1070–73.

Taylor, D. P., Carter, R. B., Eison, A. S., et al. 1995. Pharmacology and neurochemistry of nefazodone, a novel antidepressant drug. *Journal of Clinical Psychiatry* 56 (suppl. 6): 3–11.

Weise, C., Fox, I., Clary, C., et al. 1991. Nefazodone in the treatment of outpatient major depression. *Biological Psychiatry* 29:3–33.

Mirtazapine (Remeron)

Bremner, J. D. 1995. A double-blind comparison of org 3770 [Remeron], amitriptyline, and placebo in major depression. *Journal of Clinical Psychiatry* 56:519–25.

deBoer, Th. 1996. The pharmacologic profile of mirtazapine [Remeron]. *Journal of Clinical Psychiatry* 57 (suppl 4): 19–25.

Richou, H., Ruimy, P., Charbaut, J., et al. 1995. A multicenter, double-blind, clomipramine-controlled efficacy and safety study of org 3770 [Remeron]. *Human Psychopharmacology* 10: 263–71.

Zivkov, M., and DeJongh, G. D. 1995. Org 3770 [Remeron] versus amitriptyline: a 6-week randomized double-blind multicentre trial in hospitalized depressed patients. *Human Psychopharmacology* 10: 173–80.

Zivkov, M., Roes, K. C. B., and Pols, A. G. 1995. Efficacy of org 3770 [Remeron] vs amitriptyline in patients with major depressive disorder: A meta-analysis. *Human Psychopharmacology* 10 (suppl 2): S135–S145.

Side Effects

Sexual

Balon, R., Yeragani, V. K., Pohl, R., et al. 1993. Sexual dysfunction during antidepressant treatment. *Journal of Clinical Psychiatry* 54:209–12.

Feiger, A., Kiev, A., Shrivastava, R. K., et al. 1996. Nefazodone versus sertraline [Zoloft] in outpatients with major depression: Focus on efficacy, tolerability, and effects on sexual function and satisfaction. *Journal of Clinical Psychiatry* 57 (suppl. 2): 53–62.

Gitlin, M. J. 1994. Psychotropic medications and their effects on sexual function: Diagnosis, biology, and treatment approaches. *Journal of Clinical Psychiatry* 55:406–13.

Hollander, E., and McCarley, A. 1992. Yohimbine treatment of sexual side effects induced by serotonin reuptake blockers. *Journal of Clinical Psychiatry* 53:207–9.

Hopkins, H. S. 1992. Antidotes for antidepressant-induced sexual dysfunction. In Gelenberg, A. G., ed., *Biological therapies in psychiatry* 15:33–36.

Jacobsen, F. M. 1992. Fluoxetine-induced sexual dysfunction and an open trial of Yohimbine. *Journal of Clinical Psychiatry* 53:119–22.

Seizures

Rosenstein, D. L., Nelson, J. C., and Jacobs, S. C. 1993. Seizures associated with antidepressants: A review. *Journal of Clinical Psychiatry* 54:289–99.

Withdrawal

Ellison, J. M. 1994. SSRI withdrawal buzz. *Journal of Clinical Psychiatry* 55:544–45.

Nausea

Bergeron, R., and Blier, P. 1994. Cisapride for the treatment of nausea produced by selective serotonin reuptake inhibitors. *American Journal of Psychiatry* 151:1084–86.

General

McElroy, S. L., Keck, P. E., and Friedman, L. M. 1995. Minimizing and managing antidepressant side effects. *Journal of Clinical Psychiatry* 56 (suppl. 2): 49–55.

Nelson, J. C. 1994. Are the SSRIs really better tolerated than the TCAs for treatment of major depression? *Psychiatric Annuals* 24:628–31.

Nierenberg, A. A., and Cole, J. O. 1991. Antidepressant adverse drug reactions. *Journal of Clinical Psychiatry* 52 (suppl.): 40–47.

Serotonin Syndrome

Sternbach, H. 1991. The serotonin syndrome. *American Journal of Psychiatry* 148:705–13.

Mania

Peet, M. 1994. Induction of mania with selective serotonin reuptake inhibitors and tricyclic antidepressants. *British Journal of Psychiatry* 164:549–50.

Stoll, A. L., Mayer, P. V., Kolbrener, M., et al. 1994. Antidepressant-associated mania: A controlled comparison with spontaneous mania. *American Journal of Psychiatry* 151:1642–45.

Bipolar Disorder

American Psychiatric Association. 1994. Practice guideline for the treatment of patients with bipolar disorder. *American Journal of Psychiatry* 151 (12, suppl.).

Bowden, C. L. 1995. Predictors of response to divalproex [Depakote] and lithium. *Journal of Clinical Psychiatry* 56 (suppl. 3): 25–30.

———, and McElroy, S. L. 1995. History of the development of valproate [Depakene and others] for treatment of bipolar disorder. *Journal of Clinical Psychiatry* 56 (suppl. 3): 3–5.

Carlson, G. A., and Goodwin, F. K. 1973. The stages of mania. *Archives of General Psychiatry* 28:221–28.

Goodwin, F. K., and Jamison, K. R. 1990. Medical treatment of manic episodes. In Goodwin, F. K., and Jamison, K. R., eds., *Manic depressive illness*, 603–29. New York: Oxford University Press.

Marangell, L. B., and Yudofsky, S. C. 1995. Developments in the treatment of bipolar disorder. *Primary Psychiatry* 2 (6): 32–41.

Small, J. G., Klapper, M. H., Milstein, V., et al. 1991. Carbamazepine [Tegretol] compared with lithium in the treatment of mania. *Archives of General Psychiatry* 48:915–21.

Solomon, D. A., Keitner, G. I., Miller, I. W., et al. 1995. Course of illness and maintenance treatments for patients with bipolar disorder. *Journal of Clinical Psychiatry* 56:5–13.

Treatment-Resistant Depression

Klein, R. G., and Wender, P. 1995. The role of methylphenidate [Ritalin] in psychiatry. *Archives of General Psychiatry* 52:429–33.

Management of patients who are nonresponders to or nontolerators of initial antidepressant therapy. 1992. *Journal of Clinical Psychiatry*, monograph 10 (1).

Nelson, J. C. 1993. Combined treatment strategies in psychiatry. *Journal of Clinical Psychiatry* 54 (suppl.): 42–49.

Nemeroff, C. B. 1991. Augmentation regimens for depression. *Journal of Clinical Psychiatry* 52 (5, suppl): 21–27.

Phillips, K. A., and Nierenberg, A. A. 1994. The assessment and treatment of refractory depression. *Journal of Clinical Psychiatry* 55 (2, suppl.): 20–26.

Zajecka, J. M., Jeffriess, H., and Fawcett, J. 1995. The efficacy of fluoxetine [Prozac] combined with a heterocyclic antidepressant in treatment-resistant depression: A retrospective analysis. *Journal of Clinical Psychiatry* 56:338–43.

General Reference

American Psychiatric Association: Diagnostic and statistical manual of mental disorders. 1994. 4th ed. Washington, D.C.: American Psychiatric Association.

Appleton, W. S. 1991. *The fifth psychoactive drug usage guide.* Memphis: Physicians Postgraduate Press.

———. 1988. *Practical clinical psychopharmacology.* 3d ed. Baltimore: Williams and Wilkins.

Beck, A. T. 1967. *Depression: Causes and treatment.* Philadelphia: University of Pennsylvania Press.

Bloom, F. E., and Kupfer, D. J., eds. 1995. *Psychopharmacology: The fourth generation of progress.* New York: Raven Press.

Hales, R. E., Yudofsky, S. C., and Talbott, J. A. 1994. *The American Psychiatric Press textbook of psychiatry.* 2d ed. Washington, D.C.: American Psychiatric Press.

Hyman, S. E., and Nestler, E. J. 1993. *The molecular foundations of psychiatry.* Washington, D.C.: American Psychiatric Press.

Janicak, P. G., Davis, J. M., Preskorn, S. H., and Ayd, F. J. 1993.

Principles and practice of psychopharmacotherapy. Baltimore: Williams and Wilkins.

Kaplan, H. I., and Sadock, B. J. 1993. *Pocket handbook of psychiatric drug treatment.* Baltimore: Williams and Wilkins.

Schatzberg, A. F., and Cole, J. O. 1991. *Manual of clinical psychopharmacology.* 2d ed. Washington, D.C.: American Psychiatric Press.

————, and Nemeroff, C. B., eds. 1995. *The American Psychiatric Press textbook of psychopharmacology.* Washington, D.C.: American Psychiatric Press.

Shader, R. I., ed. N.d. *Manual of psychiatric therapeutics.* 2d ed. Boston: Little, Brown.

Index